Botulinum Toxin

Procedures in Cosmetic Dermatology

Series Editor: Jeffrey S. Dover MD FRCPC

Associate Editor: Murad Alam MD

Botulinum Toxin
Alastair Carruthers MABM BCh FRCPC FRCP(Lon) and Jean Carruthers MD FRCS(C) FRC(OPHTH)
ISBN 1 4160 2470 0

Soft Tissue Augmentation
Jean Carruthers MD FRCS(C) FRC(OPHTH) and Alastair Carruthers MABM BCh FRCPC FRCP(Lon)
ISBN 1 4160 2469 7

Cosmeceuticals
Zoe Diana Draelos MD
ISBN 1 4160 0244 8

Laser and Lights: Volume 1
Vascular • Pigmentation • Scars • Medical Applications
David J. Goldberg MD JD
ISBN 1 4160 2386 0

Laser and Lights: Volume 2
Rejuvenation • Resurfacing • Hair Removal • Treatment of Ethnic Skin
David J. Goldberg MD JD
ISBN 1 4160 2387 9

Photodynamic Therapy
Mitchel P. Goldman MD
ISBN 1 4160 2360 7

Liposuction
C. William Hanke MD MPH FACP and Gerhard Sattler MD
ISBN 1 4160 2208 2

Treatment of Scars
Kenneth A. Arndt MD

Chemical Peels
Mark Rubin MD

Hair Restoration
Dowling B. Stough MD and Robert S. Haber MD

Leg Veins
Tri H. Nguyen MD

Blepharoplasty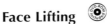
Ronald L. Moy MD

Face Lifting
Ronald L. Moy MD

PROCEDURES IN COSMETIC DERMATOLOGY

Series Editor: Jeffrey S. Dover MD FRCPC

Associate Editor: Murad Alam MD

Botulinum Toxin

Edited by

Alastair Carruthers MABM BCh FRCPC FRCP(Lon)
Clinical Professor, Division of Dermatology, University of British Columbia, Carruthers Dermatology
Center Inc., Vancouver, BC, Canada

Jean Carruthers MD FRCS(C) FRC(OPHTH)
Clinical Professor, Department of Ophthalmology, University of British Columbia, Vancouver, BC, Canada

Series Editor

Jeffrey S. Dover MD FRCPC
Associate Professor of Clinical Dermatology, Yale University School of Medicine, Adjunct Professor of
Medicine (Dermatology), Dartmouth Medical School, Director, SkinCare Physicians of Chestnut Hill,
Chestnut Hill, MA, USA

Associate Editor

Murad Alam MD
Chief, Section of Cutaneous and Aesthetic Surgery, Department of Dermatology, Northwestern
University, Chicago, IL, USA

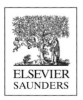

ELSEVIER
SAUNDERS

ELSEVIER
SAUNDERS

An imprint of Elsevier Inc.
© 2005, Elsevier Inc. All rights reserved.
First published 2005

ISBN: 1 4160 2470 0

British Library Cataloguing in Publication Data
A catalogue record for this book is available from the British Library

Library of Congress Cataloging in Publication Data
A catalog record for this book is available from the Library of Congress

---

Notice

Medical knowledge is constantly changing. Standard safety precautions must be followed, but as new research and clinical experience broaden our knowledge, changes in treatment and drug therapy may become necessary or appropriate. Readers are advised to check the most current product information provided by the manufacturer of each drug to be administered to verify the recommended dose, the method and duration of administration, and contraindications. It is the responsibility of the practitioner, relying on experience and knowledge of the patient, to determine dosages and the best treatment for each individual patient. Neither the Publisher nor the editor assumes any liability for any injury and/or damage to persons or property arising from this publication.

The Publisher

Printed in China
Last digit is the print number : 9 8 7 6 5 4 3 2 1

Commissioning Editors: **Sue Hodgson, Shuet-Kei Cheung**
Project Development Managers: **Martin Mellor Publishing Services Ltd, Louise Cook**
Project Managers: **Naughton Project Management, Cheryl Brant**
Illustration Manager: **Mick Ruddy**
Design Manager: **Andy Chapman**
Illustrators: **Richard Prime, Tim Loughhead**

Contents

Series Foreword
Procedures in Cosmetic Dermatology

While dermatologists have been procedurally inclined since the beginning of the specialty, particularly rapid change has occurred in the past quarter century. The advent of frozen section technique and the golden age of Mohs skin cancer surgery has led to the formal incorporation of surgery within the dermatology curriculum. More recently technological breakthroughs in minimally invasive procedural dermatology have offered an aging population new options for improving the appearance of damaged skin.

Procedures for rejuvenating the skin and adjacent regions are actively sought by our patients. Significantly, dermatologists have pioneered devices, technologies and medications, which have continued to evolve at a startling pace. Numerous major advances, including virtually all cutaneous lasers and light-source based procedures, botulinum exotoxin, soft-tissue augmentation, dilute anesthesia liposuction, leg vein treatments, chemical peels, and hair transplants, have been invented, or developed and enhanced by dermatologists. Dermatologists understand procedures, and we have special insight into the structure, function, and working of skin. Cosmetic dermatologists have made rejuvenation accessible to risk-averse patients by emphasizing safety and reducing operative trauma. No specialty is better positioned than dermatology to lead the field of cutaneous surgery while meeting patient needs.

As dermatology grows as a specialty, an ever-increasing proportion of dermatologists will become proficient in the delivery of different procedures. Not all dermatologists will perform all procedures, and some will perform very few, but even the less procedurally directed amongst us must be well-versed in the details to be able to guide and educate our patients. Whether you are a skilled dermatologic surgeon interested in further expanding your surgical repertoire, a complete surgical novice wishing to learn a few simple procedures, or somewhere in between, this book and this series is for you.

The volume you are holding is one of a series entitled "Procedures in Cosmetic Dermatology." The purpose of each book is to serve as a practical primer on a major topic area in procedural dermatology.

If you want make sure you find the right book for your needs, you may wish to know what this book is and what it is not. It is not a comprehensive text grounded in theoretical underpinnings. It is not exhaustively referenced. It is not designed to be a completely unbiased review of the world's literature on the subject. At the same time, it is not an overview of cosmetic procedures that describes these in generalities without providing enough specific information to actually permit someone to perform the procedures. And importantly, it is not so heavy that it can serve as a doorstop or a shelf filler.

What this book and this series offer is a step-by-step, practical guide to performing cutaneous surgical procedures. Each volume in the series has been edited by a known authority in that subfield. Each editor has recruited other equally practical-minded, technically skilled, hands-on clinicians to write the constituent chapters. Most chapters have two authors to ensure that different approaches and a broad range of opinions are incorporated. On the other hand, the two authors and the editors also collectively provide a consistency of tone. A uniform template has been used within each chapter so that the reader will be easily able to navigate all the books in the series. Within every chapter, the authors succinctly tell it like they do it. The emphasis is on therapeutic technique; treatment methods are discussed with an eye to appropriate indications, adverse events, and unusual cases. Finally, this book is short and can be read in its entirety on a long plane ride. We believe that brevity paradoxically results in greater information transfer because cover-to-cover mastery is practicable.

Most of the books in the series are accompanied by a high-quality DVD, demonstrating the procedures discussed in that text. Some of you will turn immediately to the DVD and use the text as a backup to clarify complex points, while others will prefer to read first and then view the DVD to see the steps in action. Choose what suits you best.

We hope you enjoy this book and the rest of the books in the series and that you benefit from the many hours of clinical wisdom that have been distilled to produce it. Please keep it nearby, where you can reach for it when you need it.

Jeffrey S. Dover MD FRCPC and Murad Alam MD

To the women in my life

My grandmothers, Bertha and Lillian
My mother, Nina
My daughters, Sophie and Isabel
And especially to my wife, Tania

For their never-ending encouragement, patience, support, love, and friendship

To my father, Mark
A great teacher and role model

To my mentor, Kenneth A. Arndt for his generosity, kindness, sense of humor, joie de vivre, and above all else curiosity and enthusiasm

At Elsevier, Sue Hodgson who conceptualized the series and brought it to reality

and

Martin Mellor for polite, persistent, and dogged determination.

Jeffrey S. Dover

The professionalism of the dedicated editorial staff at Elsevier has made this ambitious project possible. Guided by the creative vision of Sue Hodgson, Martin Mellor and Shuet-Kei Cheung have attended to the myriad tasks required to produce a state-of-the-art resource. In this, they have been ably supported by the graphics team, which has maintained production quality while ensuring portability. We are also deeply grateful to the volume editors, who have generously found time in their schedules, cheerfully accepted our guidelines, and recruited the most knowledgeable chapter authors. Finally, we thank the chapter contributors, without whose work there would be no books at all. Whatever successes are herein are due to the efforts of the above, and of my teachers, Kenneth Arndt, Jeffrey Dover, Michael Kaminer, Leonard Goldberg, and David Bickers, and of my parents, Rahat and Rehana Alam.

Murad Alam

Preface

Botulinum toxin has revolutionized the world of cosmetic procedures. When we first presented this topic in 1991, our work was greeted with some skepticism. The benefits were underrated, the risk of complications exaggerated, and the need for repeated treatments appeared a significant obstacle. Now the use of botulinum toxin is the most commonly performed cosmetic procedure in the world. Enormous expansion has occurred in the past few years in the amount of the scientific information available, the range of suitable indications, and especially the number of properly controlled studies. In this volume, we attempt to summarize this information.

With botulinum toxin being so widely used and having achieved a permanent place in the world of cosmetic procedures, we understand its esthetic effects much better. In addition, botulinum toxin has improved our understanding of facial anatomy and how the muscles of facial expression work together. The basic science has advanced in tandem with the clinical use and this is also discussed in this book. Much of this volume is ordered by anatomic areas so that the intended and unintended effects of botulinum toxin can be considered from a regional standpoint. Of course, in many faces, multiple areas are treated at the same time and botulinum toxin is increasingly used in conjunction with other procedures. Botulinum toxin is also appropriate for so-called "medical" purposes that also have a cosmetic effect; these indications, include treatment of hyperhidrosis and management of pain syndromes like headaches. Fortunately, as evidence and experience has accumulated, these have only served to confirm the low level of adverse events and the few long term risks associated with botulinum toxin use.

We anticipate that this volume will be of interest to all physicians who use or are interested in using botulinum toxin for cosmetic indications. We are most grateful to our contributing authors and our senior editors for the great amount of effort that they have collectively expended to produce a book which we trust you, the reader, will find both valuable and entertaining.

Alastair Carruthers and Jean Carruthers

List of Contributors

Murad Alam MD
Chief, Section of Cutaneous and Aesthetic Surgery, Department of Dermatology, Northwestern University, Chicago, IL, USA

Kenneth A. Arndt MD
Co-Director, SkinCare Physicians of Chestnut Hill, Chestnut Hill, MA, USA; Clinical Professor of Dermatology, Yale University School of Medicine, New Haven, CT, USA; Adjunct Professor of Medicine (Dermatology), Dartmouth Medical School, Hanover, NH, USA; Clinical Professor of Dermatology, Harvard Medical School, Boston, MA, USA

Kenneth Beer MD FAAD
Voluntary Associate Professor, University of Miami; Director, Palm Beach Esthetic Center, Palm Beach, FL, USA

Brian Biesman MD FACS
Assistant Clinical Professor, Vanderbilt University Medical Center, Nashville; Associate Clinical Professor, University of Tennessee Health Sciences Center, Memphis, TN, USA

Andrew Blitzer MD DDS
Professor of Clinical Otolaryngology, College of Physicians and Surgeons, Columbia University; Director, New York Center for Voice and Swallowing Disorders; Medical Director, New York Center for Clinical Research, NY, USA

Andres Boker MD
Director of Clinical Research, Fredric Brandt, MD PA, Coral Gables, FL, USA

Frederic Brandt MD
Private Practice, Coral Gables, FL and New York, NY, USA

Alastair Carruthers MABM BCh FRCPC FRCP(Lon)
Clinical Professor, Division of Dermatology, University of British Columbia, Vancouver, BC, Canada

Jean Carruthers MD FRCS(C) FRC(OPHTH)
Clinical Professor, Department of Ophthalmology, University of British Columbia, Vancouver, BC, Canada

Sue Ellen Cox MD
Medical Director of Aesthetic Solutions; Clinical Assistant Professor, Department of Dermatology, University of North Carolina, NC, USA

J. Charles Finn MD
Assistant Consulting Professor of Surgery, Duke University; President, Aesthetic Solutions, Chapel Hill, NC, USA

Timothy C. Flynn MD
Clinical Professor, Department of Dermatology, University of North Carolina, Chapel Hill, NC, USA

Richard G. Glogau MD
Clinical Professor of Dermatology, University of California Medical Center, San Francisco, CA, USA

Aamir Haider MD PharmD
Dermatology Resident, University of Toronto, ON, Canada

Jeffrey T.S. Hsu MD
Director of Vein Treatment Center, SkinCare Physicians of Chestnut Hill, Chestnut Hill, MA, USA

Anna Krishtul MD
Resident, Department of Medicine, University of Medicine and Dentistry of New Jersey, Springfield, NJ, USA

Nicholas J. Lowe MD FRCP
Clinical Professor, University of California School of Medicine, Los Angeles, CA, USA; Consultant Dermatologist, Cranley Clinic, London, UK; Clinical Research Specialist, Santa Monica, CA, USA and London, UK

Brent R. Moody MD
Assistant Professor of Medicine, Director of Cosmetic Dermatologic Surgery, Vanderbilt University School of Medicine, Nashville, TN, USA

Thomas E. Rohrer MD
Clinical Associate Professor of Dermatology, Boston University School of Medicine; Director of Mohs Fellowship, SkinCare Physicians of Chestnut Hill, Chestnut Hill, MA, USA

Roberta D. Sengelmann MD
Assistant Professor, Dermatology and Otolaryngology; Director, Center for Dermatologic and Cosmetic Surgery, Washington University School of Medicine, St Louis, MO, USA

Kevin C. Smith BA BsC MD
FRCPC FACP
Director, Niagara Falls Dermatology and
Skin Care Centre Ltd, Niagara Falls,
ON, Canada

Nowell Solish MD FRCPC
Assistant Professor of Dermatology,
University of Toronto, ON, Canada

Stephen R. Tan MD FRCPC
Director of Dermatologic Surgery,
HealthPartners Medical Group and
Clinics, Minneapolis, MN, USA

Stacey Tull MD MPH
Dermatology Chief Resident, Division of
Dermatology, Washington University, Saint
Louis, MO, USA

Heidi A. Waldorf MD
Associate Clinical Professor, Mount Sinai
School of Medicine; Director of Laser and
Cosmetic Dermatology, Department of
Dermatology, Mount Sinai Medical Center,
New York, NY, USA

1

Botox Esthetics

Stephen R. Tan, Richard G. Glogau

'Wrinkles should merely indicate where smiles have been'

Mark Twain, 1897

Introduction

Over the past few years, the art and science of cosmetic surgery have evolved to enable physicians to treat the signs of facial aging more precisely. In a broad sense, wrinkles may develop as either hyperdynamic lines caused by the repetitive movement of underlying facial musculature over the years, or as redundant skin which develops as the skin progressively loses its elasticity and submits to the relentless pull of gravity. For many years, the face lift and the brow lift have been the *sine qua non* of treating the wrinkles associated with inelastic and redundant skin; however, hyperdynamic wrinkles remained difficult to treat.

With the selective chemical denervation of facial musculature possible with botulinum toxin, physicians have expanded their therapeutic armamentarium to be able to treat the underlying cause of hyperdynamic lines effectively. In 1987, Drs Jean and Alastair Carruthers noticed the smoothing effect of botulinum toxin on the glabellar brow furrow when treating a patient for blepharospasm. They pursued their observations on the cosmetic effectiveness of botulinum toxin, and in 1992 published the first manuscript on the cosmetic use of botulinum toxin A (BTX-A) for treating glabellar frown lines. This observation began a new era in minimally invasive cosmetic surgery, and in 2003 they published a textbook on the subject.

To achieve maximal cosmetic improvement using botulinum toxin while minimizing the risk of complications, the physician must have a thorough understanding of facial esthetics. The word *aesthetic* is derived from the Greek word *aisthesis*, which means having a sense or love of that which is beautiful. In a modern sense, esthetics is a scientific attempt to explain a subjective concept by assigning proportions to various components of the face. The idealized face tends to exhibit several general characteristics, with slightly different proportions and shapes between women and men. Although these proportions may be used to define the 'ideal', 'attractive', or 'perfect' face, the real value in studying these principles lies in clarifying the range of normal relationships that exist between facial units. Harmony and balance of the face exist through a wide range of sizes, shapes, and configurations of the individual parts. The cosmetic surgeon must appreciate this in order to understand the changes that affect the face over time.

Etiology of the Aging Face

The face ages in response to a number of factors, which may appear to varying degrees between individuals. Sun exposure and smoking tend to accelerate these changes.

Chronic ultraviolet light damage to the skin

Photoaging adds to the inevitable changes seen with intrinsic chronologic aging; indeed, cumulative sun exposure is the single largest factor involved in our clinical perception of aging skin, and is responsible for a large portion of the unwanted esthetic effects. Glogau has developed a systematic classification of patient photoaging types (see Box 1.1 and Fig. 1.1). For a full description, please see the chapter entitled 'Filler esthetics' in the Soft Tissue Augmentation volume in this series.

Glogau photoaging classification

Type 1 – "No wrinkles"
- Early photoaging
  - Mild pigmentary changes
  - No keratoses
  - Minimal wrinkles
- Younger patient – twenties or thirties
- Minimal or no makeup

Type II – "Wrinkles in motion"
- Early to moderate photoaging
  - Early senile lentigines visible
  - Keratoses palpable but not visible
  - Parallel smile lines beginning to appear lateral to mouth
- Patient age – late thirties or forties
- Usually wears some foundation

Type III – "Wrinkles at rest"
- Advanced photoaging
  - Obvious dyschromia and telangiectasias
  - Visible keratoses
  - Wrinkles even when not moving
- Patient age – fifties or older
- Always wears heavy foundation

Type IV – "Only wrinkles"
- Severe photoaging
  - Yellow-gray color of skin
  - Prior skin malignancies
  - Wrinkled throughout, no normal skin
- Patient age – sixth or seventh decade
- Can't wear makeup – "cakes and cracks"

(Adapted from Glogau RG 1994 Chemical peeling and aging skin. Journal of Geriatric Dermatology 2(1):5–10 and Glogau RG 1996 Aesthetic and anatomic analysis of the aging skin. Seminars in Cutaneous Medicine and Surgery 15(3):134–138)

Box 1.1 Glogau photoaging classification

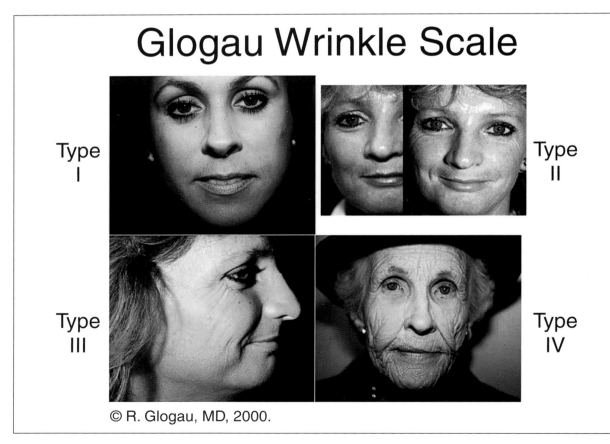

Glogau Wrinkle Scale

Type I

Type II

Type III

Type IV

© R. Glogau, MD, 2000.

Fig. 1.1 Glogau photoaging classification. In type I patients, note the absence of wrinkles and pigmentary alterations. Type II patients do not have wrinkles while the face is at rest, but wrinkles appear with facial movement. Type III patients have wrinkles present while the face is at rest. In type IV patients, the skin is entirely wrinkled, with no normal skin remaining on the face. Also note the yellow-gray, sallow color of the skin

Loss of subcutaneous fat

In general, with age there is a loss of the fullness and roundness of the facial contours of youth, resulting in a flattened or sunken appearance to facial structures.

Changes in the intrinsic muscles of facial expression and their influence on the skin

The muscles of facial expression are unique in that they insert directly into the skin. Years of facial expressions constantly folding the skin result in the progressive development of hyperdynamic wrinkles, which initially appear only with facial movement, but may ultimately remain as wrinkles at rest. Hyperdynamic wrinkles are more prominent in areas where the underlying muscles and fascia have more direct attachments to the skin, such as in the frontal, glabellar, periocular, nasolabial, and perioral areas.

Gravitational changes from loss of elasticity of the tissue

With aging, the facial soft tissues lose their inherent resiliency and ability to resist stretching; inevitably, they begin to sag under the effects of gravity.

Remodeling of the underlying bony and cartilaginous structures

Over time, bony resorption may result in a decrease in apparent facial volume, and gravitational stretch of cartilaginous structures may result in the drooping of structures such as the nasal tip. Facial asymmetry due to underlying bony or cartilaginous structural changes is difficult to correct, and pointing out these differences at the initial consultation is important in setting realistic patient expectations.

Anatomic Approach to the Aging Face

Physicians should approach a patient seeking cosmetic improvement of the signs of aging from an anatomic standpoint. The determination of *what* is wrong must precede *how* it should be corrected. All too often, physicians develop a preference for one or a few cosmetic techniques, and then attempt to apply these to all situations. Inappropriately using a therapeutic technique that does not address the underlying anatomic basis for a cosmetic problem leads to mediocre results at best, and disasters at

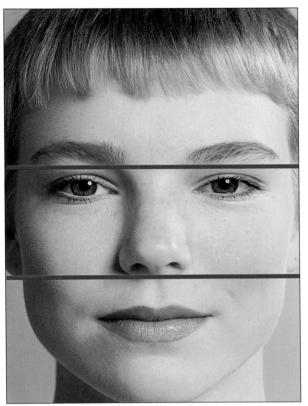

Fig. 1.2 Division of the face into thirds. The upper third ranges from the trichion to the glabella, the middle third from the glabella to the subnasale, and the lower third from the subnasale to the menton

worst. For example, patients with deep glabellar furrows treated with filler substances may experience transient improvement; however, unless the underlying muscles causing these hyperdynamic lines are paralyzed with botulinum toxin, the wrinkles will rapidly recur. Thus, an anatomic approach to the aging face is essential, and will allow the physician to rationally select the optimal therapeutic tool from a wide variety of therapeutic options.

To appreciate facial symmetry and balance, one commonly used practice is to divide the face horizontally into thirds (see Fig. 1.2). The upper third ranges from the trichion to the glabella, the middle third from the glabella to the subnasale, and the lower third from the subnasale to the menton. Botulinum toxin is mainly used to treat wrinkles in the upper third of the face, although it is being increasing utilized to treat hyperdynamic lines elsewhere.

Upper third of the aging face

Changes in the upper third of the face are primarily related to chronic ultraviolet light damage, to the intrinsic muscles of facial expression and their influence on the skin, and to gravitational changes from the loss of elasticity of the tissue. The widespread use of botulinum toxin for selective chemical denervation of facial musculature has emphasized the influence that these underlying muscles have on the skin. The forehead is undergoing constant dynamic stress from the frontalis, corrugator, and procerus muscles. These muscles are constantly active in facial expression, and convey frowning, scowling, surprise, and numerous other emotional states (see Box 1.2). Medial and lateral brow function independently in this regard, and surgeons must be aware of the strong impact that brow position can have on appearance.

The muscles of facial expression attach into the overlying dermis through the supramuscular fascia to the interlobular subcutaneous septae. Hyperdynamic wrinkles tend to develop in a direction perpendicular to the tension vector of the muscle groups; thus, the vertically oriented frontalis muscle fibers cause horizontally oriented wrinkles and furrows (see Fig. 1.3). In elderly patients with considerable actinic exposure, these transverse forehead wrinkles become crosshatched with secondary vertical creases, known as 'sleep creases'. Sleep creases result from external compression of actinically damaged skin, as opposed to the muscular etiology of hyperdynamic wrinkles (see Fig. 1.4). The corrugator muscles attach from below the orbicularis at the level of the eyebrow to the periosteum of the glabella at the nasal process of the frontal bone. Contraction produces both vertically and obliquely oriented glabellar wrinkles. Fibers

Relationship of emotional states with brow position			
Medial brow up	**Medial brow down**	**Lateral brow up**	**Lateral brow down**
Expectant	Concern	Surprise	Disdain
Quizzical	Stern	Elation	Anxious
Curious	Unhappy	Happy	Sadness
Anticipatory	Anger	Approval	Disapproval
Friendly	Fatigue		Fatigue
Serene	Mystified		
Knowing			

Box 1.2 Relationship of emotional states with brow position

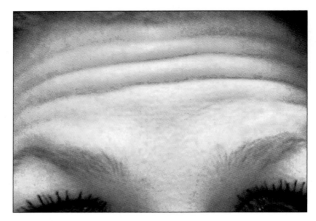

Fig. 1.3 Horizontally oriented hyperdynamic wrinkles on the forehead develop from frontalis muscle contraction

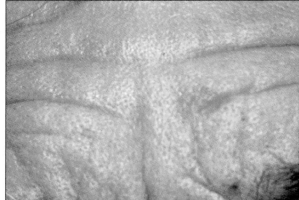

Fig. 1.4 Resting forehead wrinkles. Note that the horizontally oriented wrinkles are hyperdynamic lines resulting from frontalis muscle contraction, whereas the vertically oriented wrinkles are 'sleep creases' resulting from external compression of actinically damaged skin

of the vertically oriented procerus muscle attach from the glabella to the nasal root, and contraction produces the horizontally oriented 'scrunch' lines (see Fig. 1.5). Loss of cutaneous elasticity with age leads to glabellar ptosis, resulting in an accentuation and deepening of these wrinkles.

The esthetically ideal position of the eyebrows varies between the genders. The medial edge of the brow should have a slight club-like configuration, with a gradual taper towards the lateral end. In men, the eyebrows are ideally positioned at or just above the supraorbital rim and are almost horizontal in shape, with only the slightest hint of an arc (see Fig. 1.6). In women, the eyebrows should be positioned above the supraorbital ridge; however, unlike the relatively horizontal eyebrows in a man, the female brow has a gentle gull-wing shape, with the lateral aspect being more elevated than the medial (see Fig. 1.7). The maximal brow elevation of the female eyebrow arch occurs at or just lateral to a line tangential and vertical to the lateral limbus. The lateral brow should end at an extension of a line beginning at the nasal ala and passing through the lateral canthus. The lateral eyebrow should frame the superolateral orbital rim, which is frequently accentuated with appropriate makeup.

Obvious brow ptosis is noted when the eyebrows fall below the level of the supraorbital ridge, result-ing in a fatigued appearance (see Fig. 1.8). Brow ptosis results from a combination of gravitational stretching of inelastic skin, atrophy of the brow fat pad, alterations in the underlying soft tissue support, and a decrease in underlying bony volume. Brow ptosis may be generalized, or may be isolated to the medial or lateral portions. The fascia underlying the brow has firm attachments over the medial one-half to two-thirds of the superior orbital rim and weaker connections laterally; thus, the weaker lateral connections allow for brow ptosis to typically be greater along the lateral aspects. Lateral brow ptosis is seen clinically as temporal hooding and, if there is concomitant upper lid ptosis, may interfere with vision. Patients may attempt to compensate by

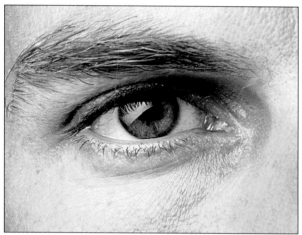

Fig. 1.6 Idealized male brow, positioned at the supraorbital rim with an almost horizontal shape

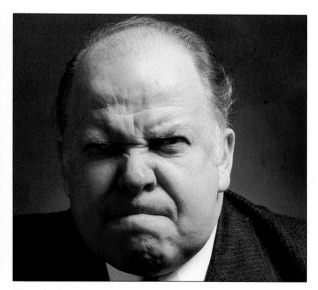

Fig. 1.5 Glabellar hyperdynamic wrinkles. Corrugator muscle contraction produces both vertically and obliquely oriented wrinkles, whereas procerus muscle contraction leads to horizontal 'squinch' lines

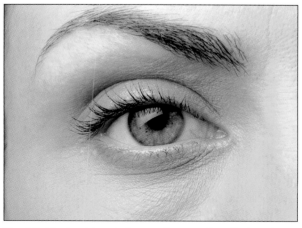

Fig. 1.7 Idealized female brow, with a gentle gull-wing shape

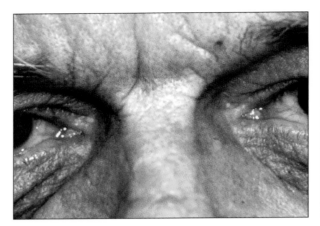

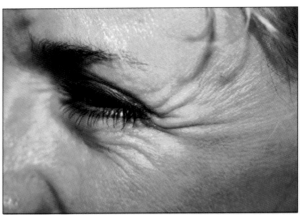

Fig. 1.8 Brow ptosis. Note brow position below the level of the supraorbital ridge, as well as early hooding as the upper eyelid skin droops towards the visual axis

Fig. 1.9 'Crow's feet' hyperdynamic wrinkles radiating outwards from the lateral canthus

cocking the head back slightly and by contracting the frontalis muscles in an attempt to raise the drooping brow, adding to the forehead furrows. This is commonly seen in males and is typically perceived as a masculine characteristic, whereas in females it may be perceived with a negative connotation.

On the lateral aspects of the face, wrinkles may develop as 'crow's feet' emanating radially from the lateral canthi (see Fig. 1.9). Analogous to the hyperdynamic wrinkles in the forehead and glabella regions, crow's feet result from the accordion-like movement of the orbicularis oculi muscles. With progressive loss of cutaneous elasticity, the skin is less able to rebound from the continued pulling of the underlying muscles, and these wrinkles may eventually remain at rest.

Middle third of the aging face

Aging of the middle third of the face affects the lower eyelids and periorbital regions, the cheeks, and the nose. Changes in these areas primarily result from a combination of photoaging, loss of subcutaneous tissue, loss of cutaneous elasticity, and remodeling of underlying cartilaginous and bony structures. For a full description of the changes in this area, please see the chapter entitled 'Fillers esthetics' in this series.

Lower third of the aging face

The age-related changes seen in the lower third of the face affect the lips, the chin, the lower cheeks,

and the neck. Changes result from a combination of chronic ultraviolet light damage to the skin, loss of subcutaneous fat, changes due to the muscles of facial expression, gravitational changes from a loss of elasticity of the tissue, and remodeling of the underlying bony and cartilaginous structures.

Wrinkles form around the lips as a result of the constant pulling of the orbicularis oris muscle on progressively more inelastic upper- and lower-lip skin, creating angular, radial, and vertical wrinkles (see Fig. 1.10). The effects of gravity result in drooping of the oral commissures laterally and downward, which may lead to a tired and sad appearance. Fullness of the lips and a strong definition of the philtrum are seen in youth; however, with advancing age there is a thinning of the vermillion, loss of lip highlights, and an overall flattening of the lip.

For a full description of the other age-related changes occurring in this area, please see the chapter entitled 'Fillers esthetics' in this series.

Conclusion

The introduction of botulinum toxin for selective chemical denervation has emphasized the impact of facial musculature on the appearance of facial aging. Complete or partial weakening of the glabellar corrugator/procerus muscle complex, the forehead frontalis, and the lateral orbicularis oculi muscles has revolutionized the management of the upper third of the aging face. Deep glabellar lines, which could only briefly be improved with injectable

An appreciation of the patient's baseline state is essential to attaining a successful cosmetic outcome. With a thorough working knowledge of facial esthetics, anatomy, and the changes seen with aging, the cosmetic surgeon can approach a patient with hyperdynamic wrinkles to effectively utilize botulinum toxin to achieve maximal cosmetic improvement.

Further Reading

Carruthers A, Carruthers J 2003 The cosmetic use of botulinum neurotoxin. Martin Dunitz, London

Dzubow L 1997 The aging face. In: Coleman WP III, Hanke CW, Alt TH, Asken S (eds) Cosmetic surgery of the skin: principles and techniques, 2nd edn. Mosby, St Louis, pp. 7–17

Gliklich RE 1997 Proportions of the aesthetic face. In: Cheney ML (ed) Facial surgery: plastic and reconstructive. Williams & Wilkins, Baltimore, MD, pp. 147–157

Glogau RG 2002 Evaluation of the aging face. In: Kaminer MS, Dover JS, Arndt KA (eds) Atlas of cosmetic surgery. WB Saunders, Philadelphia, pp. 29–33

Glogau RG 2003a Botulinum toxin. In: Freedberg IM, Eisen AZ, Wolff K, Austen KF, Goldsmith LA, Katz SI (eds) Fitzpatrick's dermatology in general medicine, 6th edn. McGraw-Hill, New York, pp. 2565–2567

Glogau RG 2003b Systematic evaluation of the aging face. In: Bolognia JL, Jorizzo JL, Rapini RP (eds) Dermatology. Mosby, London, pp. 2357–2360

Hanke CW 2002 The history of cosmetic dermatologic surgery. In: Kaminer MS, Dover JS, Arndt KA (eds) Atlas of cosmetic surgery. WB Saunders, Philadelphia, pp. 18–28

McKinney P, Cunningham BL 1992a Anatomy. In: McKinney P, Cunningham BL (eds) Aesthetic facial surgery. Churchill Livingstone, New York, pp. 25–51

McKinney P, Cunningham BL 1992b Midface. In: McKinney P, Cunningham BL (eds) Aesthetic facial surgery. Churchill Livingstone, New York, pp. 77–91

McKinney P, Cunningham BL 1992c Upper face. In: McKinney P, Cunningham BL (eds) Aesthetic facial surgery. Churchill Livingstone, New York, pp. 53–76

Powell N, Humphreys B 1984 Proportions of the aesthetic face. Thieme-Stratton, New York

Ridley MB, VanHook SM 2002 Aesthetic facial proportions. In: Papel ID, Frodel J, Park SS, Holt GR, Sykes JM, Larrabee WF, et al (eds) Facial plastic and reconstructive surgery, 2nd edn. Thieme, New York, pp. 96–109

Salasche SJ, Bernstein G, Senkarik M 1988 Surgical anatomy of the skin. Appleton & Lange, Norwalk, CT

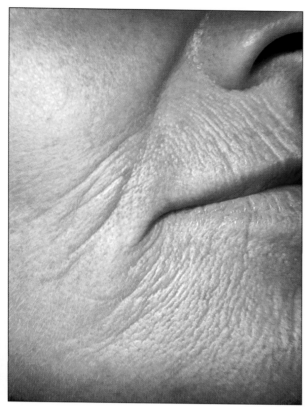

Fig. 1.10 Perioral wrinkles radiating outward from the upper and lower lips. 'Marionette lines' form as vertical wrinkles extending downwards from the oral commissures

fillers, are now effectively treated with the placement of botulinum toxin in the procerus and corrugator muscles and orbicularis oculi. Crow's feet lines, which routinely reappeared 2–3 months after deep resurfacing, now vanish after a few days. Even troublesome horizontal lines and creases of the lower eyelid that persist after blepharoplasty and/or resurfacing can be treated with botulinum toxin.

2

Background to Botulinum Toxin

Thomas E. Rohrer, Ken Beer

Introduction

Every time a patient walks into your office and says 'Doc, I don't want that poison injected into my body,' the history of botulinum toxin collides with your daily life. Botulinum toxin has gone from a deadly disease and a highly secretive biologic weapons program to something that is talked about (and, in some parts of the USA, administered) over cappuccino. The story of this transformation is quite interesting.

History

Botulism is a form of food poisoning that usually begins as blurred vision, dry mouth, dizziness, and nausea that may progress to deadly, flaccid paralysis. Early outbreaks were believed to be caused by sausage, thus the name was derived from the Greek word for sausage, *botulus*. Although botulism was well known in historical legend, the modern story of botulinum toxin began with a Belgian picnic in 1895 that went bad. At that picnic, 34 people became ill after eating raw salted ham. Three of them later died due to progressive paralysis. The etiologic agent was identified by Professor Emile Pierre Marie van Ermengem and named *bacillus botulinus*; it was reclassified later as *Clostridium botulinum*. It is an anaerobic, spore-forming bacterium that, under the proper conditions, can germinate and create a toxin. He noted that the toxin produced was not heat-resistant, but did hold against alcohol, enzymes, and mild acid. He also noted that although some animals responded similarly to humans, some, such as chickens and dogs, were seemingly unaffected by the toxin.

With these findings, van Ermengem hypothesized what we now know to be true of the botulinum toxins:

- botulism is an intoxication, not an infection
- the toxin is produced by something in food
- the toxin is relatively resistant to mild chemical agents but very susceptible to heat
- the toxin is produced in food of high salt concentration
- not all species react in the same manner to the toxin.

The process of isolation and development of the toxins began in 1920 by Dr Herman Sommer. Type A toxin was isolated in 1946 by Edward Shantz for the US Army and, in 1949, Burgen discovered the mechanism by which the toxin functioned. Although type A strains are responsible for the majority of human cases of botulism, types B and E have also been documented as the causative strains.

Medical use of botulinum toxin (BTX) began in the 1950s with Dr Vernon Brooks and was significantly advanced in the 1970s by Dr Alan Scott. The first study demonstrating therapeutic value for BTX-A was published in 1973. This study showed that injections of BTX-A could weaken extraocular muscles in monkeys. It took until 1977 before the treatment was attempted in humans. Dr Shantz prepared the first batch of what came to be called 'Botox' in 1979. This tiny 150 mg batch, labeled 11-79, served as the source of all BTX-A used in humans in the USA up until 1997. Since December 1997, a Food and Drug Administration (FDA)-approved BTX-A source has been used (Allergan Inc., Irvine, CA). Dr Scott's original company, Oculinum Inc., was acquired by Allergan Inc. in 1989 and the name of the product was changed to 'Botox'.

In 1979, the FDA granted limited approval to use BTX-A for strabismus and, in 1985, this was expanded to include blepharospasm. In 1989, the FDA approved the use of Allergan's BTX-A for strabismus, blepharospasm, and hemifacial spasm. In 2003, it was approved for the treatment of glabellar rhytides.

The lack of approval for specific indications did not hurt BTX-A usage and it was tried for nystagmus, torticollis, spasmodic dystonia, and many other diseases related to muscle dysfunction. A 1999 *New England Journal of Medicine* editorial entitled 'One Man's Poison – Clinical Applications of Botulinum Toxin' provides examples of the various historic uses of BTX such as relieving lower limb spasticity to allow children to walk or permitting movement of the upper arms so that children can wash themselves. Among the more unusual (and successful) uses for BTX was the treatment of anal fissures.

In 1987, while treating patients for benign essential blepharospasm, Dr Jean Carruthers made the magical observation that led to today's most popular cosmetic procedure. She noted that many of the patients being treated for blepharospasm with BTX had significant improvement of dynamic rhytides in the glabellar region. Following this observation, Drs Alastair and Jean Carruthers initiated more systematic studies of BTX for cosmetic usage. The Carruthers reported initial findings of cosmetic treatment with BTX in 1991 and published their findings in a seminal paper in 1992, demonstrating the safe and effective treatment of dynamic rhytides in the glabella with BTX-A. In 1993, Blitzer and colleagues described the use of BTX for rhytides of the forehead and elsewhere.

Subsequent usage and publications by physicians such as Drs Arnold Klein, Nicholas Lowe, Patricia Wexler, Richard Glogau, Steven Fagien, and numerous others expanded the usage of BTX. New areas for treatment such as the platysma, crow's feet, and hyperhidrosis were demonstrated to be safe and effective.

Mirroring the expanded indications for cosmetic usage, the therapeutic indications for BTX have also increased. Among the new therapeutic uses which have grown out of the cosmetic use is the treatment of headaches and migraines.

Physiology

Most facial rhytides form perpendicular to the direction of underlying muscular contractions. As skin loses its elasticity with age and photoaging, it does not rebound as well from the constant forces of stress placed upon it, and wrinkles form. A good

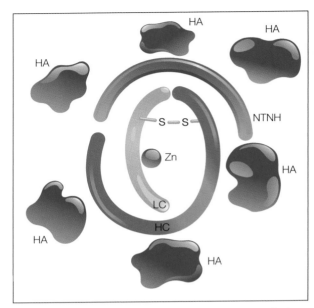

Fig. 2.1 Illustration of the large 900 kDa botulinum toxin A structure. Note that the actual botulinum toxin itself only makes up 150 kDa of the structure, the rest is made up of large protective hemagglutinin and nonhemagglutinin proteins. The complex is held together by noncovalent bonds that are stable in the acidic environment of the gastrointestinal tract but dissociate as the pH increases in the blood stream and release the free toxin

example of this is the pattern of horizontally oriented lines on the forehead. Forehead rhytides form perpendicular to the vertically contracting frontalis muscle. When the facial muscles responsible for creating the wrinkles are not functionally necessary, BTX may be injected to temporarily paralyze or weaken them and ameliorate the lines.

As interest in Botox increased, so did our knowledge of how it functions. *C. botulinum* bacteria produces seven serologically distinct types of botulinum neurotoxin (designated as types A, B, C1, D, E, F, and G). All subtypes of botulinum neurotoxin act by preventing the release of acetylcholine at the neuromuscular junction of striated muscle fibers, creating a flaccid paralysis of the muscle. Of the known subtypes of BTX, type A appears to be the most potent in humans and was the first one available in a commercial formulation (Botox, Allergan Inc. and Dysport, Ipsen, Inc. Berkshire, UK). The toxin exists in its native state complexed with nontoxic proteins. In fact, the toxin itself only makes up 150 kilodaltons (kDa) of the total 900 kDa molecular weight of the BTX-A complex structure (Fig. 2.1). The remainder of the structure is made

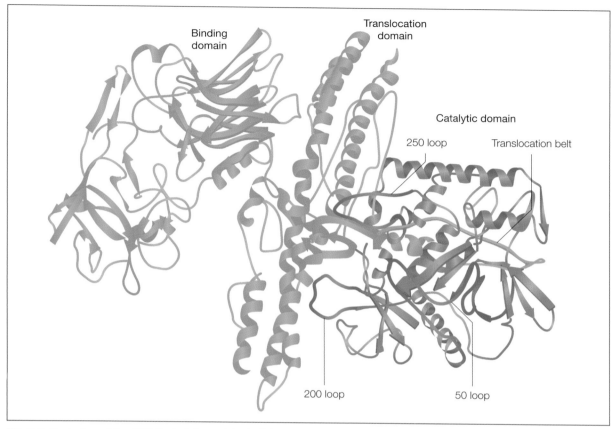

Fig. 2.2 Illustration of the 150 kDa botulinum A toxin. It is comprised of a 100 kDa heavy chain (responsible for the high affinity, irreversible, docking on the presynaptic nerve membrane) on the left and a 50 kDa light chain (responsible for the cleavage of proteins in the synaptic fusion complex) on the right. The heavy and light chains are held together by a disulfide bond

up of large protective proteins, primarily hemagglutinins, held together by covalent bonds that are very stable in acidic environments. This clever structure serves to protect the ingested toxin in the harsh acidic environment of the gut. As the toxin goes out into the bloodstream and the pH rises, the bonds dissociate and the free neurotoxin is released to have its effect on striated muscles.

The BTX molecule is a 150 kDa structure made up of a 100 kDa heavy chain and a 50 kDa light chain held together by a disulfide bond and associated with a zinc atom (Fig. 2.2). The heavy chain has the C-terminus on it and is responsible for the high affinity docking on the presynaptic nerve membrane (Fig. 2.3). This binding is rapid and irreversible. *In vitro*, it can be adjusted to occur in approximately 32–64 min. The light chain is responsible for the intracellular cleavage of proteins required for transmission of acetylcholine across

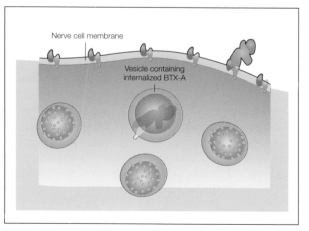

Fig. 2.3 Illustration of the botulinum toxin molecule bound to the presynaptic nerve membrane and another botulinum toxin molecule internalized into the cytosol of the nerve ending. The C-terminus located on the heavy chain is responsible for the rapid and irreversible binding on the membrane

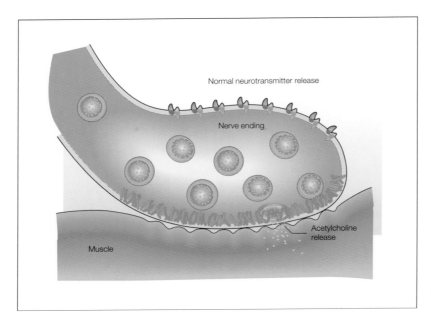

Normal neurotransmitter release

Nerve ending

Acetylcholine
release

Muscle

Fig. 2.4 Illustration of the preformed
vesicles of acetylcholine in the
presynaptic motor nerve ending

the neuromuscular junction (NMJ). The different
subtypes of BTX have unique areas on the nerve
membrane to which they bind and have different
proteins within the presynaptic nerve terminal
that they cleave. However, they all have the same
mechanism of action; to act as a zinc-dependent
endoprotease and inhibit the release of the neurotransmitter acetylcholine at the peripheral NMJ,
leading to a flaccid paralysis.

In a normal nerve ending at the NMJ, there exist
numerous small preformed vesicles containing
the neurotransmitter acetylcholine. As an action
potential travels down a nerve and reaches the nerve
ending, it causes the vesicles to dock to the terminal
membrane of the junction (Fig. 2.4). The membranes
fuse and acetylcholine from the vesicles is released
into the synaptic cleft. Acetylcholine is bound to the
postsynaptic muscle and a muscular contraction is
initiated. What allows the preformed acetylcholine
vesicles to dock and fuse to the membrane is a
structure termed the synaptic fusion complex.
The synaptic fusion complex is made up of a group
of proteins known as the SNARE (soluble *N*-
ethylmaleimide-sensitive factor attachment protein
receptors) proteins (Fig. 2.5).

Two sets of SNARE proteins exist and are
required for fusion and neurotransmitter release:
one on the acetylcholine containing vesicle and
another group on the neuronal membrane. The set
on the vesicle is known as the v-SNARE or
the vesicular SNARE proteins VAMP-2 (vesicle-
associated membrane protein-2) and the two on the
target membrane are known as t-SNAREs. In the
cytoplasm, vesicular (v-)SNARE VAMP-2 engages
with two plasma membrane t-SNAREs, syntaxin 1A
and SNAP-25 (synaptosome-associated protein of
25 kDa), to form the crucial heterotrimer core
complex that bridges the two membranes and
allows for neurotransmitter release. Another
protein, MUNC18-1, has also been theorized to
play a role in the fusion of the vesicle and membrane. The process is fundamentally triggered by
calcium influx in response to an action potential
and may be regulated by the N-terminal α-helical
domain of syntaxin 1A. Release of the neurotransmitter occurs very rapidly. It is estimated to
happen in less than 0.5 ms after calcium influx. It
has been proposed that SNARE core complex
formation proceeds like a zipper, from the membrane distal end toward the membrane proximal
end. The SNARE complex formation is an energy-
releasing process that may supply the required free
energy for membrane fusion.

This SNARE core complex is the location of
action for botulinum toxins. If one or more of the
SNARE proteins are damaged, the acetylcholine
vesicles are not able to dock and fuse and acetylcholine will not be released. This results in a

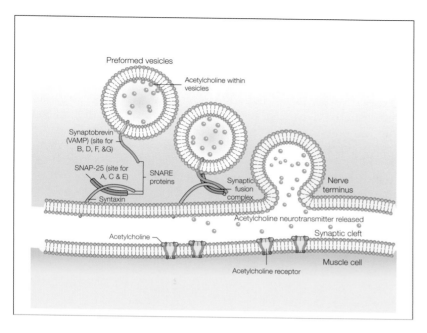

Preformed vesicles

Acetylcholine within vesicles

Synaptobrevin (VAMP) (site for B, D, F, &G)

SNAP-25 (site for A, C & E)

SNARE proteins

Syntaxin

Synaptic fusion complex

Nerve terminus

Acetylcholine neurotransmitter released

Acetylcholine

Synaptic cleft

Acetylcholine receptor

Muscle cell

Fig. 2.5 Close up illustration of the SNARE proteins in the synaptic fusion complex at the neuromuscular junction. Botulinum toxins A, C, and E catalyze the cleavage of the SNAP-25 protein. Botulinum toxins B, D, F, and G catalyze the cleavage of synaptobrevin (or the vesicle-associated membrane protein, VAMP)

paralysis of that particular associated muscle cell. For more detailed information on this complex subject, see the further reading at the conclusion of this chapter.

After the heavy chain of BTX has bound to the outer membrane of the terminal nerve at the NMJ, it is internalized into the cytoplasm of the nerve cell through receptor cell-mediated endocytosis. Internalization is dependent on energy and temperature, and is accelerated by nerve stimulation. As the newly formed vesicle enters the nerve cell's cytosol, it contains both the heavy and light chain of the BTX held together by the disulfide bond. Soon the light and heavy chains dissociate and the light chain is released into the nerve cytoplasm. The light chain then travels to the junction and catalyzes the cleavage of SNARE proteins in the synaptic fusion complex. The light chains of botulinum toxins A, C, and E catalyze the cleavage of SNAP-25 (synaptosomal-associated protein), a 25 kDa protein of the SNARE complex. The light chains of botulinum toxins B,D, F, and G catalyze the cleavage of a different SNARE protein in the synaptic fusion complex known as synaptobrevin or the VAMP. Type C may also cleave syntaxin. Either way, the synaptic fusion complex is inactivated and the presynaptic vesicles cannot dock, fuse, and release their acetylcholine, the neurotransmitter. Although striated muscle NMJs are most sensitive to the toxin, autonomic cholinergic nerves, for example those responsible for sweat production, and also nosioreceptors are affected by BTX.

Botulinum toxin does not damage the nerve or alter the production of acetylcholine. Only the structure responsible for the transmission of the signal across the NMJ is damaged. Once the synaptic transmission is inhibited, the target structures no longer function. In the case of skeletal muscle, this means contraction ceases. Clinically, muscle weakness is seen approximately 2–4 days following injection, with full paralysis or maximal weakness complete at 7–10 days. The time to onset and maximal efficacy differs among BTX products and may be dose-dependent, with more rapid onset following higher doses. Over time, the terminal nerve ending begins to form new smaller unmyelinated nerve endings, termed peripheral sprouts. Peripheral sprouting begins to occur within 28 days and activity returns to the nerve muscle complex in approximately 3 months. Peripheral sprouts may originate from the terminal node of Ranvier, the unmylinated terminal axon just retrograde to the end plate, or the terminal axon site itself. Although it was originally thought that the peripheral sprouting resulted in new normal NMJs, recent evidence suggests that the SNAP-25 proteins eventually regenerate in the original NMJ and re-establish the initial connection. The peripheral sprouts then retract over time and disappear. Muscles paralyzed by BTX-A return to function approximately 2–5 months after injection, depending on the dose administered. Repeated injections are typically performed at this interval to keep facial rhytides from reforming.

When skeletal muscle is repeatedly treated with Botox, some degree of atrophy may be demonstrated. This may result in treatments that require less units of toxin as well as treatments that may occur at increased time intervals.

It is also these authors' observation that patients retain some improvement of their dynamic rhytides for more than a year even without repeat treatment. Patients returning 1–2 years following a single BTX injection often have rhytides that are not as deep by photographic evaluation as they were before their initial treatment. One explanation for this is that, because there is less collagen at the depth of an active rhytide, allowing the area to rest for a period of time may give the body the opportunity to deposit more collagen in the depth of the rhytide.

Most drugs are measured and administered by their weight, typically in the milligram range. However, the amount of toxin used in medical treatment with BTX is so small that it must be measured in terms of its biologic activity rather than by its mass. The dose of BTX, usually in the nanogram range (10^{-9}), is measured in units of biologic activity in a standardized mouse model. One unit of biologic activity, commonly referred to as 1 unit, is the amount of toxin required to kill 50% (lethal dose or LD_{50}) of 18- to 20-g female Swiss-Webster mice when injected intraperitoneally. The estimated lethal dose in a 100 kg human is approximately 3500 times this, or 3500 units. In the standardized mouse model, 1 unit of Botox will have the same effect as 1 unit of Myobloc, which will have the same effect as 1 unit of Dysport. There is, however, significant species variation and this same one-to-one relationship does not cross over to other species. When comparing Botox (BTX-A) to Myobloc (BTX-B) the 1:1 relationship seen in the mouse model changes to approximately 1:5 in the Cynomolgus monkey hand model, and may be between 1:125 and 1:150 in the treatment of dynamic rhytides of the glabellar region in humans. More studies are looking into the differences between BTX-A and BTX-B and the use of a simple conversion factor between the two may not turn out to be the best way to use and evaluate BTX-B.

Botulinum toxin has also been advocated for use in the treatment of hyperhidrosis. When BTX is injected intradermally, it inhibits acetylcholine release from cholinergic nerve fibers associated with eccrine and apoeccrine sweat glands and thus reduces or eliminates the production of sweat from the treated glands. Palmar, plantar, axillary, and facial hyperhidrosis have all been successfully treated with BTX injections. Duration of action against hyperhidrosis is considerably longer than that seen with the treatment of dynamic rhytides. Anhidrosis following BTX has been reported to last between 4 and 12 months.

Storage, Handling, and Dilution

BTX-A is commercially available in North America as BOTOX (Allergan Inc.). It comes in a vial containing 100 units of BTX-A in lyophilized form (Fig. 2.6). The vial contains approximately 5 ng of the neurotoxin and a small amount of sodium chloride (0.9 mg) and human albumin (0.5 mg) added as a stabilizer. Although the vials have always contained 100 units of the toxin, originally the vials were manufactured with approximately 25 ng of the

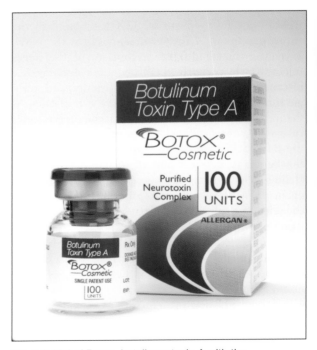

Fig. 2.6 Vial of Botox, botulinum toxin A with the unreconstituted product seen as the small white ring of powder seen around the base of the vial. Vial contains 100 units of botulinum exotoxin A in lyophilized form, as well as a small amount of sodium chloride (0.9 mg) and human albumin (0.5 mg)

toxin protein, much of which was inactive. Because antibody formation and subsequent resistance to the toxin has been linked to the total cumulative neurotoxin protein dose, decreasing the protein dose to one-fifth the original dose should decrease the risk of antibody formation and resistance. It should be noted that, to date, with an estimated over 5 million injections, there are no known cases of antibody formation and resistance to BTX when doses typically employed for the cosmetic treatment of dynamic rhytides are used. Resistance is, however, seen in neurologic patients being treated with doses in the 100 and 200 unit range. Patients receiving large and frequent doses of BTX seem to be at the highest risk for the formation of neutralizing antibodies. Because there is no significant crossreactivity between the different subtypes of BTX, it may be possible to treat a patient that has become resistant to BTX-A with BTX-B.

The vial of Botox has traditionally been kept frozen (–5°C) until used. However, new evidence suggests that there is no significant change in the shelf life or efficacy of Botox if it is stored in a refrigerator rather than a freezer.

Additionally, the manufacturer recommends that Botox be reconstituted with 0.9% sterile, preservative-free saline, a recent report suggests that reconstituting the lyophilized toxin with saline preserved with benzyl alcohol 0.9% may decrease pain during injection by as much as 54% without altering the efficacy. Benzyl chloride is known to have some anesthetic effect. When patients were injected with Botox reconstituted with preservative-free saline on one side and preserved saline on the other, none chose the side with preservative-free saline as being less painful.

The amount of saline used to reconstitute BTX varies widely between practitioners. Placing anywhere between 1 and 10 mL of saline into the 100 unit vial, with corresponding dilutions of 100 to 10 units/mL, have been published. Although this has been a somewhat controversial point for several years, recent studies suggest within the range of 0.2–10 units/0.1 cc, there was no noted difference in efficacy or degree of action. They did, however, note greater diffusion with lower concentrations (higher dilutions). These authors recommend finding a dilution and remaining consistent with it. Botulinum toxin injections should be thought of and discussed in terms of units and not in terms of volume. This will help reduce confusion and potential over- or under-dosing.

Many early articles and textbook chapters have stated that the crystalline complex of the high molecular weight BTX protein and hemagglutinin may be easily denatured by shaking or allowing bubbles to percolate through the solution during or following reconstitution. This led to the recommendation of being extremely gentle in the handling of BTX. Recent reports have found no statistical difference in efficacy between Botox that had been gently handled and Botox that had been shaken and foamed during reconstitution for at least 4 months following injection.

The manufacturer of Botox recommends using the product within 4 hours of reconstitution. This recommendation is mandated by the FDA for any product reconstituted with preservative-free saline and is for sterility issues and not a loss in efficacy. As to how long Botox is fully potent after reconstitution remains somewhat controversial. Gartland and Hoffman noted significant loss of toxicity at 12 hours after reconstitution, and Lowe noted a 50% decrease in potency after 1 week. However, Garcia and Fulton reported continued potency 4 weeks after reconstitution. In a recent controlled study with 88 patients, Hexsel found no statistically significant difference in efficacy or duration of action between bottles of Botox that had been reconstituted at the time of the injection, 2 weeks, 4 weeks, and even 6 weeks prior to injection.

Myobloc™ (BTX-B) comes as a solution in vials of 2500, 5000, and 10 000 units. BTX-B is less potent than BTX-A in humans and Myobloc requires approximately 50–150 times the dose of Botox to achieve similar results in dynamic rhytides. Myobloc is reported to be more stable than Botox and may be kept refrigerated at 2–8°C for up to 21 months. It is noteworthy that all of the commercially available neurotoxins are labeled indicating that they should be discarded if the contents are not used within 4 hours of reconstitution/broaching the vial.

Resistance to Chemodenervation

Resistance to chemodenervation with any of the botulinum toxins is rare. It is believed that the development of resistance to treatment is due to production of blocking antibodies. As with other immunologic events, the production of antibodies depends on the immune system of the host as well as the immunogenicity of the stimulus.

The older, functional Botox literature reports blocking antibodies in approximately 5% of patients treated for cervical dystonia. However, these patients were treated with the original lot of Botox which had a higher protein content (25 ng/vial)than does the present lot (5 ng/vial).

Despite the increasing popularity of Botox for cosmetic usage, the rate of blocking antibodies appears to be quite low. The rate of patients that are nonresponders is even lower because patients that develop antibodies may still have a clinical response to Botox. According to Allergan, only 1–2% of patients will develop antibodies to Botox and the correlation of these antibodies to clinical response is not clear.

The factors that are the most important in the development of blocking antibodies are the dose per session and the interval between the dose. The cumulative dose does not appear as important as these two factors. Patients treated with high doses (300 units of Botox or higher) at frequent intervals seem the most likely to develop antibodies to Botox. Cosmetic patients treated with Botox typically utilize 25–75 units at intervals of several months and are not very likely candidates to develop resistance. In addition, it seems unlikely that cosmetic patients that require small doses (2–10 units) of Botox as a 'touchup' following a treatment will have a significant risk of developing antibodies.

For patients that are resistant to chemodenervation with one subtype of BTX, a trial with a different subtype is indicated. In addition, an attempt should be made to measure antibodies to determine if the resistance is antibody mediated. Because there are several different toxins available, resistance to one subtype does not preclude treatment with another.

Summary

All eight of the known subtypes of botulinum neurotoxin act as zinc-dependent endoproteases and prevent the release of acetylcholine at the NMJ of striated muscle fibers causing a flaccid paralysis. Of the known subtypes of botulinum toxin, type A is the most potent in humans, and was the first one available in a commercial formulation (Botox, Allergan Inc., Irvine, CA). When facial muscles responsible for creating unwanted rhytides are not functionally necessary, minute doses of BTX may be injected to temporarily paralyze or weaken the muscles and ameliorate the lines. Botox, BTX-A, is manufactured and distributed in a lyophilized form, which is reconstituted using saline, with or without preservative. The reconstituted Botox is fairly stable and very likely may be used for several weeks following reconstitution with minimal loss of potency. Myobloc, BTX-B, is distributed in solution form of various concentrations and may be used for up to 2 years without significant loss of potency.

Botulinum toxin injections are now reported to be the most common cosmetic procedure performed in this country. Although the results are not long term, BTX injections provide outstanding clinical results for a variety of facial rhytides with almost no recovery time. As our population continues to seek less invasive treatments for the signs of aging, the use of BTX is likely to continue to rise.

Further Reading

Alam M, Dover JS, Arndt KA 2002 Pain associated with injection of botulinum toxin A exotoxin reconstituted using isotonic sodium chloride with and without preservative: a double-blind, randomized controlled trial. Archives of Dermatology 138(4):510–514

Bushara KO, Park DM, Jones JC, Schutta HS 1996 Botulinum toxin: a possible new treatment for axillary hyperhidrosis. Clinical and Experimental Dermatology 21:276–278

Carruthers A, Carruthers JA 1992 Treatment of glabellar frown lines with C. Botulinum A exotoxin. Journal of Dermatological Surgery in Oncology 1S:17–21

Carruthers A, Carruthers J 2000 Toxins 99, new information the botulinum neurotoxins. Dermatological Surgery 26:174–176

Carruthers J, Carruthers A 1996 Cosmetic uses of botulinum A exotoxin. In: Dzubow L (ed) Advances in Dermatology 12:280–303

Carruthers JDA, Strubbs HA 1987 Botulinum toxin for benign essential blepharospasm, hemifacial spasm and age-related lower eyelid entropion. Canadian Journal of Neurological Science 14:42–45

de Paiva A, Ashton AC, Foran P, et al 1993 Botulinum A like type B and tetanus toxins fulfills criteria for being a zinc-dependent protease. Journal of Neurochemistry 61:2338–2341

Goschel H, Wohlfarth K, Frevert J, et al 1997 Botulinum A toxin therapy: neutralizing and nonneutralizing antibodies – therapeutic consequences. Experimental Neurology 147:96–102

Hallett M 1999 One man's poison – clinical applications of Botulinum toxin. New England Journal of Medicine 341:118–120

Hexsel D, De Almeida T, Rutowitsch M, et al 2003 Multicenter, double-blind study of the efficacy of injections with botulinum toxin type A reconstituted up to six consecutive weeks before application. Dermatological Surgery 29:523–529

Jankovic J, Schwartz K 1995 Response and immunoresistance to botulinum toxin injections. Neurology 45:1743–1746

Kaminer MS, Hruza GJ 2002 Botulinum A exotoxin injections for photoaging and hyperhidrosis. In: Cosmetic surgery procedures and techniques. WB. Saunders, Philadelphia, pp.291–294

Klein A 2003 Botulinum toxin complications. Dermatological Surgery 29:549–556

Kweon DH, Kim CS, Shin YK 2003 Regulation of the neuronal SNARE assembly by the membrane. Nature Structural Biology 10(6):440–447

Lowe NJ 1998 Botulinum A toxin type A for facial rejuvenation: United States and United Kingdom perspectives. Dermatological Surgery 24:1216–1218

Pearce LB, Borodic GE, First ER, et al 1994 Measurement of Botulinum toxin activity: evaluation of the lethality assay. Toxicology and Applied Pharmacology 128:69–77

Rizo J, Sudhof T 2002 SNARES and MUNC-18 in synaptic vesicle fusion. Nature Reviews 3:641–652

Schiavo G, Benfenati F, Poulain B, et al 1992 Tetanus and botulinum B neurotoxins block neurotransmitter release by proteolytic cleavage of synaptobrevin. Nature 359:832–835

Scott AG 1981 Botulinum toxin injection of eye muscles to correct strabismus. Transactions of the American Ophthalmology Society 79:734–740

Setler P 2000 The biochemistry of botulinum toxin B. Neurology 55(12, suppl 5):S22–S28

Simpson LL 1986 Molecular pharmacology of botulinum toxin and tetanus toxin. Annual Reviews in Pharmacological Toxicology 26:427–453

Spencer JM 2002 Botulinum toxin B: the new option in cosmetic injection. Journal of Drugs in Dermatology 1:17–22

Trinidad De Almeida AR, Kadunc BV, Di Chiacchio N, et al 2003 Foam during reconstitution does not affect the potency of botulinum toxin type A. Dermatological Surgery 29:530–532

Practical Botulinum Toxin Anatomy

3

J. Charles Finn, Sue Ellen Cox

Introduction

Effective and precise use of botulinum toxin type A (BTX-A) demands comprehensive understanding of facial anatomy. Detailed understanding of muscle location is vital to beginning a botulinum toxin practice, but the true artist will have developed a much deeper understanding of origins, insertions, vectors of pull, and anatomic variation. Continual study and restudy of anatomic research will advance every treating physician's precision in treatment of complex patients. Physicians should take every opportunity to advance their knowledge through preceptorships and, most importantly, cadaver study.

We will describe relevant anatomy important in chemodenervation as well as methods to understand anatomic and functional variation. Anatomic variation has often been neglected in classical anatomy texts. Sometimes anatomic misconceptions are propagated through the years from text to text. We will attempt to clarify several anatomic variations as well as ways to understand anatomy through physical examination of the patient. Although this chapter is far from exhaustive, it does serve as an essential springboard towards further anatomic study.

Anatomy

The upper third

The influence of the eyebrows is crucial in establishing appearance, mood, and facial expression. In females, the eyebrow should arch gracefully above the supraorbital rim and should lie about 1 cm above the orbital rim, with the highest point directly above the lateral limbus. The position of the male brow is at the superior orbital rim and is more flat. With aging, the lateral brow descends, making the female brow more masculine. The shape of the brows can be greatly influenced by BTX chemodenervation.

Placement of BTX can produce either medial or lateral brow elevation or depression, dramatically affecting facial expression.

The eyebrows provide a foundation of support for the lids and represent an area in which the frontalis and orbicularis muscles interdigitate. The frontalis muscle is the sole elevator of the eyebrow. There are four eyebrow depressor muscles: procerus, corrugator supercilii, depressor supercilii, and orbicularis oculi. These fibers intermingle and are difficult to separate at their cutaneous insertions. The muscles in the superficial plane include the frontalis, procerus, and the orbicularis oculi; deeper muscles include corrugator supercilii, procerus, and depressor supercilii. To understand fully the anatomy of this region, one must also understand the changing depth of these muscles. For example, the corrugator begins deep medially, and becomes more superficial as it extends laterally, finally having dermal insertions (Fig. 3.1).

Frontalis

The vertically oriented frontalis muscle elevates the eyebrow. The frontalis muscle originates on the galea aponeurotica at various levels along the coronal suture and inserts on the dermis at the level of the eyebrow, interdigitating with fibers of the procerus, corrugator, and orbicularis oculi muscles. There is no bony insertion for the frontalis muscle. Classical anatomy texts usually depict the frontalis as a muscle with two distinct and separate bellies (Fig. 3.2A). In browlift surgery, most surgeons note a predominance of a single, broad expanse of muscle (Fig. 3.2B).

There are two functional muscle patterns seen clinically. The more common pattern reveals single contiguous transverse forehead lines (Fig. 3.2D). Dissection in these patients shows a broad band of frontalis muscle without separation. The second pattern seen more commonly in anatomy texts,

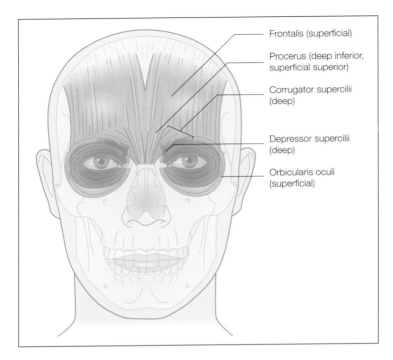

Fig. 3.1 Forehead musculature

Labels:
- Frontalis (superficial)
- Procerus (deep inferior, superficial superior)
- Corrugator supercilii (deep)
- Depressor supercilii (deep)
- Orbicularis oculi (superficial)

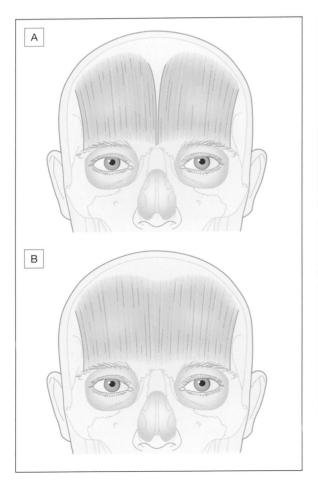

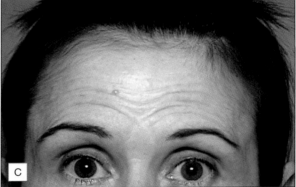

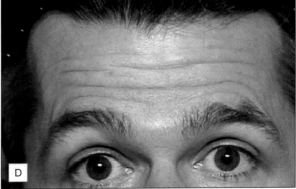

Fig. 3.2 (**A**) Classic frontalis description, two muscle bellies. (**B**) Frontalis more common configuration with broad muscle. (**C**) Patient with separate muscle bellies – no muscle in midline. (**D**) Patient with more common single frontalis muscle

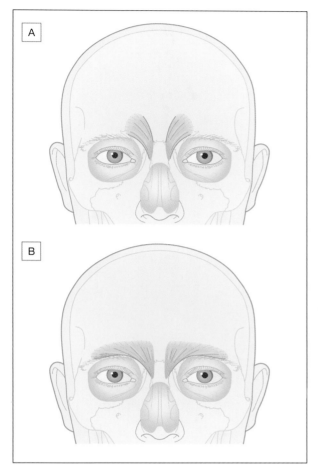

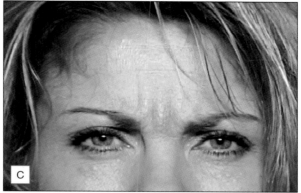

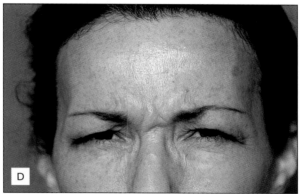

Fig. 3.3 (**A**) Short, square corrugator pattern. (**B**) Broad, flat corrugator pattern. (**C**) Clinical short, square corrugator. (**D**) Clinical broad, flat corrugator. Note lateral dimple with contraction

but less common clinically, shows two broad bands of frontalis muscle with a central separation. In patients with two separate muscle bellies, two distinct arches are noted above each brow (Fig. 3.2C). At times, the central forehead is smooth while the lateral forehead is corrugated.

Corrugator supercilii muscle

Contraction of the corrugator supercilii muscle (CSM) adducts and slightly depresses the eyebrow, moving it inferiorly and medially. Repetitive contraction produces the vertical or oblique glabellar creases. The CSM is deep centrally, extending more superficial laterally. It originates from the medial supraorbital ridge of the frontal bone. The origin has a wide base, and cadaver dissections show the origin of the CSM compartmentalized into three or four thin, rectangular, pane-like sheets of muscle. The muscle groups travel in parallel, running obliquely in a lateral and superior direction. The insertion of the CSM occurs gradually, interdigitating with the frontalis muscle and inserting in the skin in the region of the midbrow. A study analyzing 50 cadaver hemibrow dissections revealed two distinct muscle patterns. The first pattern showed a short, narrow pyramidal muscle located at the medial end of the supraorbital ridge (Fig. 3.3A). The second pattern had a long narrow, straight muscle extending along the supraorbital ridge to or beyond the midbrow position (Fig. 3.3B). These different patterns are easily visible clinically (Figs 3.3C and 3.3D). As the patients contract the corrugator complex, a skin dimple is visible at the skin insertion. Injections should follow the anatomical course of the muscle. For vertical glabellar rhytides, BTX-A injections should be into the thickest portion of the CSM adjacent to the medial aspect of the brow and even

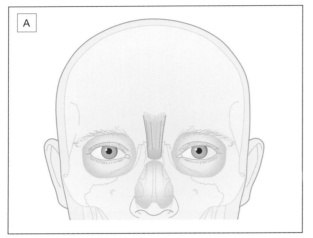

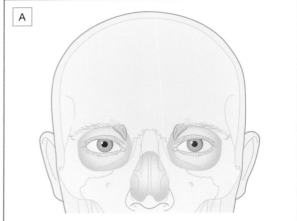

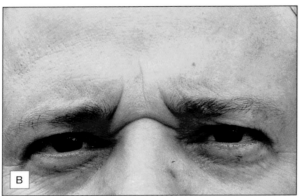

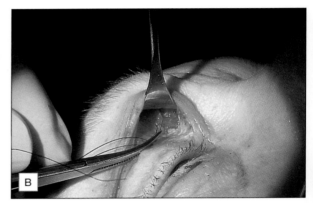

Fig. 3.4 A) Procerus. **(B)** Procerus hyperfunction pattern

Fig. 3.5 (A) Depressor supercilii. **(B)** Intraoperative identification of depressor supercilii

with or above the horizontal plane passing through the eyebrow. If the lateral corrugator is missed, some mid to lateral brow furrowing will still be visible with contraction. This may be corrected with additional treatment in the superficial, lateral portion of the muscle.

Procerus

The procerus muscle is a thin, narrow brow depressor muscle (Fig. 3.4A). It draws the medial aspect of the eyebrows down, producing transverse wrinkles over the nasal bridge (Fig. 3.4B). The origin of the procerus muscle is the periosteum of the nasal bone. Insertion is into the glabellar or mid forehead dermis. For horizontal rhytides over the nasal bridge, the procerus muscle should be injected in the midline, slightly caudal to the root of the nose.

Depressor supercilii muscle

The depressor supercilii muscle (DSM) is a brow depressor that originates from the nasal portion of the frontal bone approximately 1 cm above the medial canthal ligament and inserts in the dermis beneath the medial head of the eyebrow (Fig. 3.5A). Controversy has surrounded the existence of this muscle. Some have suggested that the DSM is a portion of the corrugator muscle, whereas others have suggested that this muscle is a portion of the orbicularis oculi muscle, or perhaps a distinct entity. The DSM may be seen surgically when the corrugator complex is approached through the upper eyelid incision (Fig. 3.5B). Cook and colleagues also isolated this distinct muscle in several cadaver specimens. Two patterns were seen: those specimens originating with two distinct heads and those with one distinct head. In those with two heads, the angular vessels passed between the two heads. In those with one head, the angular vessels were anterior to the muscle. The transverse head of the CSM is superior and medial to the DSM. Knowledge of this depressor muscle will allow one to effectively inactivate it with BTX. The injection should be either subcutaneous or slightly deeper in a vertical line extending from 10 to 15 mm above the medial canthal tendon.

Orbicularis oculi

The orbicularis oculi is a broad sphincteric muscle with copious dermal insertions. Indeed, this muscle is intimately associated with the very thin eyelid dermis and is surgically very difficult to separate from the overlying eyelid skin. The orbicularis has its bony origins near the medial canthus. The effects of orbicularis contraction vary depending on the location in the orbit. BTX treatment is directed to specific portions of this muscle for a variety of effects.

In the upper and lower lid, the muscle is divided into three portions, although the orbicularis anatomically appears as a single sheet (Fig. 3.6A). The orbicularis is divided into pretarsal, preseptal, and orbital portions. Each of the divisions originates at the medial canthal tendon or the medial orbital bone. Laterally, the pretarsal and preseptal sections insert at the lateral canthal tendon. The orbital portion loops around the lateral canthal tendon without inserting. Laterally, there is a broad expanse of vertically oriented fibers, the transition from horizontal to vertical occurring at the temporal fusion line.

The medial/superior portion of the orbicularis oculi acts as a medial brow depressor. This portion of the orbicularis is superficial to the small depressor supercilii and lateral to the procerus. The origins are on the nasal process of the frontal bone near the medial canthus and the insertions are spread over the dermis of the upper lid and brow. BTX treatment of this portion of the muscle will elevate the medial brow.

The upper orbicularis acts as a brow adductor, and can be quite active in chronic 'squinters'. Often, there is a vertical crease in the mid-brow in such individuals. This crease can be difficult to treat with BTX. Treatment of this line requires a superficial treatment of the orbicularis inferior to the brow, which places the patient at risk for eyelid ptosis.

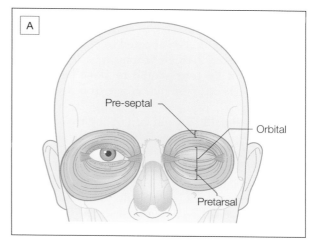

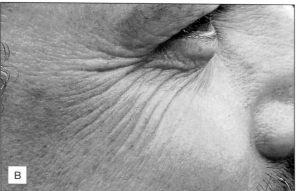

Fig. 3.6 (**A**) Orbicularis oculi. (**B**) Crow's feet from lateral orbicularis oculi hyperfunction

The lateral corrugator muscle pierces and interdigitates with the orbicularis between the mid-pupilary line and the lateral canthus.

Laterally, the orbicularis oculi acts as a lateral brow depressor, and treatment of the lateral muscle can elevate the brow to some degree. The lateral orbicularis is of course also responsible for 'crow's feet,' and exhibits excellent response to treatment (Fig. 3.6B). The extent of the lateral orbicularis varies considerably among patients. Treatment generally follows the contour and extent of the crow's feet.

As the inferior lateral orbicularis fibers curve more medially, the muscle becomes an accessory elevator of the cheek. If this area is aggressively treated to 'chase' rhytides, a flattening of the malar area becomes evident. This may present as a deepening of the nasojugal fold.

The horizontal portion of the inferior orbicularis is a crucial support mechanism of the lower eyelid.

The tarsal portion of the orbicularis should be treated cautiously with BTX. This treatment needs to be a low dose and would be expected to open the ocular aperture and smooth hypertrophic muscle. A careful assessment of lid tone should be done before this treatment, as ectropion may result from weakening of a lax lid.

Caution should be exercised in the treatment of the inferior preseptal orbicularis. The orbital septum restrains the orbital fat, which is often psuedo-herniated. This condition may be congenital or due to an age-related change. The preseptal orbicularis supports the septum, specifically during smiling. If the septal orbicularis is weakened, the lower lids may appear swollen, creating a look of fatigue. Some physicians feel this swelling is also due to an excess of lymphatic fluid. The septal orbicularis is also thought to play a role in the 'pumping' of lymphatic fluid.

The orbital and medial portion of the orbicularis may become more evident following treatment of the lateral orbicularis muscle. A medial inferior angular rhytide may be seen with smiling which may be treated with a small dose of BTX.

Chemodenervation of the orbicularis oculi muscle is accomplished with very superficial subdermal or intradermal injections. Superficial injections limit bruising and decrease deep diffusion, while allowing a controlled lateral diffusion.

Midface anatomy

The midface presents anatomical challenges for the average clinician. The muscular structure is complex and variable (Fig. 3.7A). The actions of individual muscles are never in isolation as each muscle has an agonist/antagonist relationship with surrounding muscles. Treatment of the middle third of the face with BTX is challenging and requires experience, detailed anatomic knowledge, and judicious dosing. However, in the properly selected patient, midface treatment can be very rewarding. Treatment can address asymmetry, the nasolabial fold, lip rhytides, and lip malposition. We will present an overview of individual muscle function in relation to chemo-denervation treatment.

Zygomaticus major

This muscle is relatively constant between patients. The zygomaticus major has its origin in the inferior aspect of the body of the zygoma, deep to the orbital orbicularis muscle. This muscle inserts in the modiolus in the corner of the mouth. One-third of cadavers demonstrate a bifid zygomaticus major muscle and, on occasion, a fascial band will extend to the dermis, contributing to a dimple (Fig. 3.7B). Contraction of the zygomaticus major muscle pulls the corner of the mouth laterally and superiorly. The zygomaticus major muscle does not significantly contribute to the formation of the nasolabial fold.

Treatment of this muscle is seldom indicated, and should be done with very low doses. The only indication for this treatment may be with severe asymmetry associated with facial nerve dysfunction or severe hemifacial spasm. If treatment of the orbicularis muscle is too deep and too inferior, the zygomaticus major may be affected. Paresis of this muscle causes a profound droop to the corner of the mouth.

Zygomaticus minor

The zygomaticus minor muscle, when present, has its origin just medial to the origin of the zygomaticus major and its insertion on the orbicularis oris medial to the modiolus. The zygomaticus minor is absent in two-thirds of cadaver dissections. This muscle may contribute to the nasolabial fold. Its function is thought to be relatively minor. There are no clear anatomic landmarks to determine the presence or absence of this muscle. Treatment is seldom indicated.

Levator labii superioris

This muscle has a wide origin on the malar bone just below the infraorbital rim, deep to the orbicularis and SOOF (suborbicularis oculi fat) and superior to the infraorbital nerve. This muscle interdigitates with the medial orbicularis and elevates the upper lip. Contraction also contributes to the midportion of the nasolabial fold. Treatment with BTX-A flattens the nasolabial fold while preventing elevation of the upper lip while smiling. Treatment is very rare, and usually indicated only for facial asymmetry.

Levator labii superioris alequae nasi

This is a long tubular muscle with origins on the nasal process of the maxilla and insertions at the medial orbicularis oris and at the nasal ala.

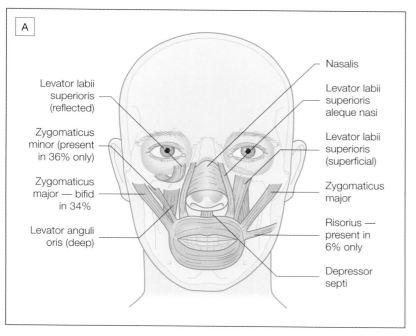

Levator labii superioris (reflected)

Zygomaticus minor (present in 36% only)

Zygomaticus major — bifid in 34%

Levator anguli oris (deep)

Nasalis

Levator labii superioris aleque nasi

Levator labii superioris (superficial)

Zygomaticus major

Risorius — present in 6% only

Depressor septi

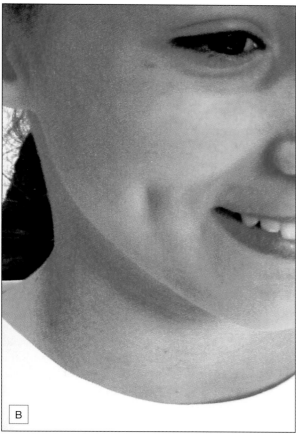

Fig. 3.7 (**A**) Midface musculature. (**B**) Dimple caused by dermal attachments of zygomaticus major

Contraction of the levator labii superioris alequae nasi has several effects. First, this muscle is a major contributor to the medial nasolabial fold, and a lesser contributor to the mid nasolabial fold. Second, this muscle serves as a lesser levator of the central lip. Third, contraction elevates the nasal ala, creating the illusion of a ptotic nasal tip during smiling. With maximal contraction, oblique lines may form on the nasal sidewall, sometimes called 'bunny lines.' Unilateral contraction creates a classic sneer.

Chemodernervation of this muscle is challenging, but can be rewarding in carefully selected patients. Very small doses of BTX placed just lateral to the piraform aperture dramatically soften the nasolabial fold, but prevent full elevation of the central portion of the lip during a smile. The best candidates for this treatment have deep folds and a gummy, canine type of smile. In these carefully selected patients, treatment has the double effect of softening the nasolabial fold and normalizing the smile. If treatment is done in patients with a normal smile, the central lip covers too much of the incisors during smiling. In some patients this change may be too different from the usual smile to justify treatment, despite an improved nasolabial fold.

Levator anguli oris

This muscle has its origin on the face of the maxilla and extends directly inferior, inserting at the modiolus. It serves to elevate the corner of the mouth, but does not contribute to the nasolabial fold. Chemodernervation is rarely indicated.

Nasalis

This muscle has two parts. The pars alaris has its origin on the face of the maxilla above the incisors and inserts on the alar cartilage. This portion dilates the nostrils. The pars transversa has its origin just superior to the pars alaris and extends in a thin expanse over the cartilaginous nasal dorsum to the contralateral ala. Contraction of this muscle pulls the ala towards the midline. Contraction of this muscle may also contribute, along with the superior portion of the levator labii superioris aleque nasi and the inferior medial portion of the orbicularis oculi, to the formation of oblique 'bunny lines.' Conservative treatment of these muscles with BTX may soften these lines.

Depressor septi

This is a small muscle with origins at the nasal spine of the maxilla and insertions on the mesial crura of the lower lateral cartilages. Contraction pulls the nasal tip downwards and slightly constricts the nostrils. In selected patients, conservative chemo-denervation may slightly elevate the nasal tip at rest. Treatment of this muscle as well as the levator labii superioris aleque nasi will help to prevent the nasal tip from pulling downward with smiling.

Lower third and neck

Like the midface, the lower third of the face is challenging to treat and requires detailed anatomic knowledge (Fig. 3.8). However, treatment of this area is very common and effective. Experienced clinicians should not shy away from treatment of this area, but should be precise and careful with treatment. Treatment can elevate the corner of a frowning mouth, smooth a dimpled chin, and relax overactive neck bands.

Orbicularis oris

This muscle is a large sphincter structure which surrounds the mouth. Contraction patterns can form complex shapes to the lips, crucial to communication and mastication. The orbicularis oris can seal the mouth, protrude the lips, or pull the lips to the teeth. There are multiple interdigitations with all other muscles of the lower face. Laterally, the orbicularis oris coalesces into a musculotendonous structure, the modiolus. Multiple facial muscles insert into the modiolus and control the corner of the mouth.

The orbicularis oris muscle is often treated with BTX to improve vertical lines of the upper and lower lips. Treatment needs to be conservative due to the vital functional nature of this muscle. Treatment should be done with small, superficial, and symmetrical doses. Even with appropriate treatment, generating a tight oral seal may be difficult. This can be noticed when drinking through a straw or when smoking. The lip may feel stiff and the patient may have a subjective sensation of dysarthria. In some cases, plosive sounds ('p' and 'b') may be impaired. The smaller doses used may have a relatively short duration of action.

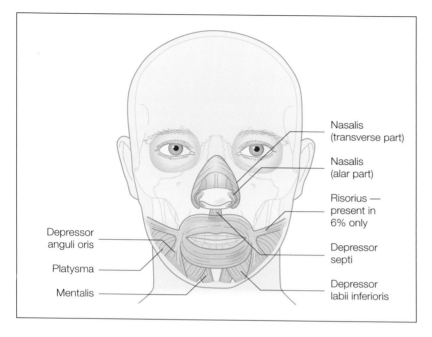

Fig. 3.8 Lower third musculature

Labels on figure:
- Nasalis (transverse part)
- Nasalis (alar part)
- Risorius — present in 6% only
- Depressor septi
- Depressor labii inferioris
- Depressor anguli oris
- Platysma
- Mentalis

Risorius

This vestigial muscle is present in only 6% of cadaver specimens. When present, this muscle extends from the preparotid fascia to the modiolus and pulls the corner of the mouth laterally. When present, this muscle parallels the superficial fibers of the platysma muscle in both form and function.

Depressor anguli oris

This superficial muscle originates from the inferior mandibular border near the mandibular ligament, a fibrous attachment between the mandible and the dermis. The depressor anguli oris inserts in the modiolus. The upper half of this muscle, with the platysma muscle, has significant dermal insertions. These dermal insertions are the cause of the labio-mandibular or chin–jowl groove. Contraction of the depressor anguli oris occurs with frowning and turns down the corner of the mouth (Fig. 3.9).

Chemodenervation of this muscle is useful in treating the aging mouth. Conservative treatment with BTX decreases the resting tone of the muscle and elevates the corner of the mouth. Treatment must be kept superficial and lateral to prevent inadvertent chemodenervation of the depressor labii inferioris. Side effects of this treatment include food trapping in the gingivolabial sulcus and subjective dysarthria. These side effects are transient and abate 3–4 weeks following treatment.

Depressor labii inferioris

This muscle originates on the mandible superior and medial to the origin of the depressor anguli oris and inserts on the inferior orbicularis oris. The depressor labii inferioris is the main depressor of the central lip. Innervation is from the marginal mandibular

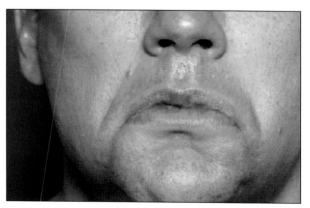

Fig. 3.9 Depressor anguli oris contraction

branch of the facial nerve, which is susceptible to injury during certain surgeries such as facelift, parotidectomy, and submandibular gland excision. If this nerve is injured, the paretic side of the lower lip is abnormally elevated during smiling. This muscle is rarely treated with BTX and usually only treated to restore facial symmetry in cases of facial nerve malfunction. Inadvertent treatment of this muscle causes a distorted smile with a high position of the lower lip, and difficulty with food trapping.

Mentalis

The mentalis is a depressor of the central chin with origins on the mentum and multiple fibrous dermal insertions. In classical anatomic texts, it is pictured as a rectangular paired muscle with oblique orientation. Practically, it is a more diffuse muscle with many small fibers extending from the periosteum of the mentum to the dermis. Contraction not only depresses the soft tissue of the chin, but creates a unique pebbly texture to the overlying skin (Fig. 3.10). This textural appearance of the chin is present throughout life, but becomes more apparent with the subcutaneous atrophy of aging. Many patients are unaware that their chin texture changes with various expressions, as this only appears with animation. When patients examine their own faces in a mirror, their face is usually in repose. When this condition is brought to the attention of the patient, they are very grateful to have effective treatment with chemodenervation. A relatively small dose of BTX-A in the chin provides a very effective smoothing. Again, care should be taken to avoid a superior

injection that would affect the depressor labii inferioris.

Platysma

The platysma is a broad, flat band of muscle with complex actions and considerable natural variation. The platysma has its origin in multiple locations on the clavicle, first rib and acromion, as well as dermal insertions in the anterior chest below the clavicles. It is a paired muscle that extends in a broad expanse over the anterior neck to the mandible. Posteriorly, the platysma runs over the mandible, but interiorly the muscle inserts on the anterior inferior mandible. The anterior portion of the platysma acts as a depressor of the mandible, but posteriorly the muscle turns interiorly and is a depressor of the corner of the mouth.

The anterior platysma has three main patterns in the neck, and much of neck aging patterns can be attributed to these platysma anatomy patterns. In 15% of patients, the platysma joins at the level of the hyoid with muscle fascicles interdigitating in a wide decussation (Fig. 3.11A). This creates an effective sling to the submental space. In the majority of patients, the bands of platysma are separate at the hyoid, but decussate a few centimeters below the insertion in the mandible (Fig. 3.11B). In 10%, the platysma never decussates and instead inserts as two separate muscles at the midline (Fig. 3.11C).

Anterior platysma bands become prominent with aging in many patients with separated platysma bands. The most dramatic neck aging is in patients with no decussation who develop a 'turkey neck' as the anterior muscle slides forward in two distinct ptotic cords (Fig. 3.11D). Surgical therapy is often directed towards uniting these bands to form a more effective submental sling. Patients with more decussated anterior platysma muscles will tend to have a better submental contour with aging.

Some patients develop several hyperfunctional bands of the platysma muscle. These are only visible in thinner patients and may become more apparent after cosmetic procedures such as facelift and submental liposuction. Hyperfunctional (as opposed to ptotic) platysmal bands may be effectively treated with BTX-A. This may be done with EMG guidance, but is more commonly treated without EMG. The key to treatment is to avoid overtreatment or treatment deep to the platysma as disastrous complications

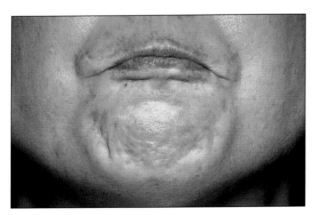

Fig. 3.10 Mentalis contraction

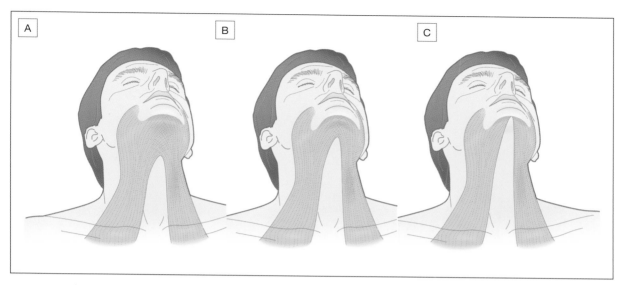

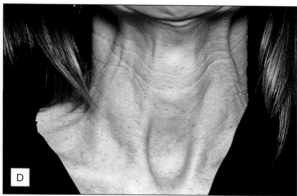

Fig. 3.11 (**A**) Platysma with complete decussation—fibers interlace from hyoid to mentum to form sling. (**B**) Platysma with partial decussation, most common pattern. (**C**) Platysma with no decussation, predisposes patient to prominent bands with aging. (**D**) Clinical photo with anterior banding from lack of decussation

have been reported with diffusion to the deeper muscles of the neck. These complications have included severe dysphagia, aspiration, and voice change.

The superior portion of the platysma is often neglected or misunderstood and also has some interesting variations. As the posterior platysma passes over the mandible it interdigitates with other muscles and fibers of the SMAS (superficial musculoaponeurotic system) and turns anteriorly to insert on the modiolus and the depressor anguli oris (Fig. 3.12A). Contraction of this portion of the muscle pulls the corner of the mouth downwards and laterally. In some patients, the platysma has considerable dermal insertions lateral to the modiolus in parallel with the nasolabial fold (Fig. 3.12B). In these patients, a smile or grimace produces a lateral crease in the skin which can be difficult to treat (Fig. 3.12C).

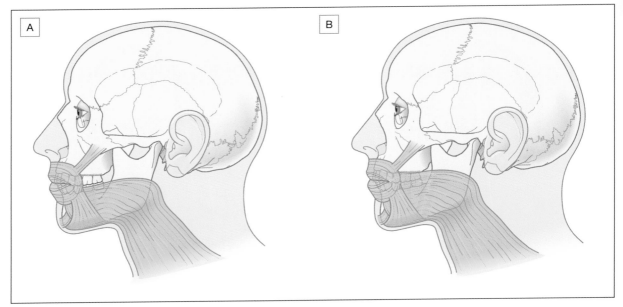

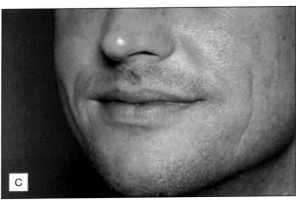

Fig. 3.12 (**A**) Platysma with classical insertion into dermis at depressor anguli oris. (**B**) Platysma with lateral insertion causing lateral facial crease. (**C**) Clinical photo of lateral facial crease from platysma dermal insertion

Further Reading

Cook BE Jr, Lucarelli MJ, Lemke BN 2001 Depressor supercilii muscle: anatomy, histology, and cosmetic implications. Opthalmological Plastic and Reconstructive Surgery 17(6):404–411

De Castro CC 1980 The anatomy of the platysma muscle. Plastic and Reconstructive Surgery 66(5):680–683

Kane M 2003 The effect of botulinum toxin injections on the nasolabial fold. Plastic and Reconstructive Surgery 112(5): 66s–72s

Knize DM 2000 The muscles that act on glabellar skin: a closer look. Plastic and Reconstructive Surgery 105(1): 350–361

Lemke BN, Stasior OG 1982 The anatomy of eyebrow ptosis. Archives of Opthamology 100:981–986

Macdonald M, Spiegel J, Raven R, et al 1998 An anatomical approach to glabellar rhytids. Archives of Otolaryngological Head and Neck Surgery 124(12):1315

Park J, Hoagland T, Park M 2003 Anatomy of the corrugator supercilli muscle. Archives of Facial Plastic Surgery 5(5):412–415

Patrinely JR, Anderson RL 1988 Anatomy of the orbicularis oculi and other muscles. Advances in Neurology 49:15–23

Pessa JE, Brown F 1992 Independent effect of various facial mimetic muscles on the nasolabial fold. Aesthetic Plastic Surgery 16(2): 167–171

Pessa JE, Garza PA, Love VM, Zadoo VP, Garza JR 1998 The anatomy of the labiomandibular fold. Plastic and Reconstructive Surgery 101(2):482–486

Pessa JE, Zadoo VP, Adrian EK, Yuan CH, Aydelotte J, Garza JR 1998 Variability of the midfacial muscles: analysis of 50 hemifacial cadaver dissections. Plastic and Reconstructive Surgery 102(6): 1888–1893

Pogrel MA, Schmidt BL, Ammar A, Perrott DH 1994 Anatomic evaluation of the anterior platysma muscle. International Journal of Oral and Maxillofacial Surgery 23(3):170–173

Shorr N, Seiff SR 1986 Cosmetic blepharoplasty: an illustrated surgical guide. Slack, Thorofare, NJ

Zufferey J 1992 Anatomic variations of the nasolabial fold. Plastic and Reconstructive Surgery 89(2):225–231

4

Upper Face Treatment

Alastair Carruthers, Jean Carruthers

Introduction

The first reports of botulinum toxin type A (BTX-A) use in the face were published in the early 1990s, although clinicians impressed with the simplicity, safety, and remarkable effects of BTX-A had been experimenting with cosmetic applications in the face since the late 1980s. Our experience with BTX-A began in 1982, and in 1987 we noted that patients treated for blepharospasm showed improvement in glabellar lines. In 1992, we published the first report detailing cosmetic use of BTX-A; around this time, other investigators described esthetic benefits in patients treated for facial dystonias. From these initial reports to the present, cosmetic use of BTX-A has grown exponentially. BTX-A is widely discussed in the popular media and the treatment is increasingly popular with patients. Its use has expanded such that BTX-A injections are now among the most commonly performed cosmetic procedures in the practice of dermatology.

The initial use of BTX-A was in the upper face. The beneficial effect on frown lines and brow position produced a very positive enhancement of facial expression and was the most obvious cosmetic response to the agent. Other areas of the face are now routinely treated with BTX-A but the upper face remains the most commonly treated area. In addition, our knowledge of the effect of BTX-A in this area has increased dramatically and this has influenced injection technique to increase further the positive appearance change and to reduce complications.

The simplicity and safety of BTX-A treatment are among its most compelling attributes, but BTX-A is nonetheless a powerful neurotoxin. Its successful use in cosmetic applications demands thorough knowledge of facial musculature (Fig. 4.1) and the action of the toxin, as well as a sound understanding of proper injection technique. This is increasingly important as the indications in which BTX-A is applied become more sophisticated and complex. In this chapter we provide an overview of the cosmetic use of BTX-A in the upper face, including preoperative considerations, injection techniques, postoperative care, optimizing outcomes, and minimizing complications.

Our clinical experience lies primarily with Botox (also known as Botox Cosmetic and Vistabel). Unless otherwise specified, all references to BTX-A in this chapter refer to the Botox, Botox Cosmetic, or Vistabel formulations.

Patients

Patient selection

Appropriate patient selection is crucial to the success of cosmetic BTX-A treatment. BTX-A is effective in subjects with negative facial signals caused by underlying muscle pull (Fig. 4.2). Individuals with deep frown lines, severe facial lentigines, telangiectasia, and telangiectatic matting with fine rhytides and diminished skin texture may not achieve a satisfactory response to BTX-A treatment alone; the overall appearance of age and fatigue may persist in such patients after treatment.

Patient education

Patient education is a crucial element of successful cosmetic BTX-A treatment. The clinician should carefully explain the procedure, the course and duration of clinical effects, the fact that repeat treatment will be necessary after 3–6 months, and possible adverse effects. The patient should be informed about what to expect following treatment, and any safety concerns should be addressed. The

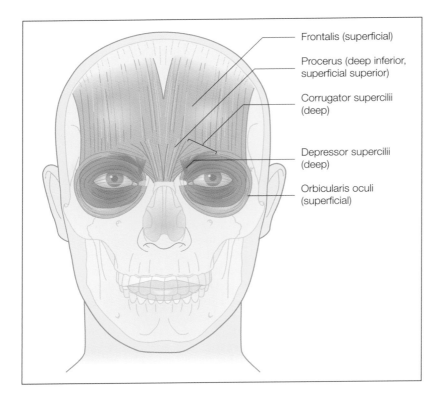

Fig. 4.1 Relevant musculature of the upper face

Frontalis (superficial)

Procerus (deep inferior, superficial superior)

Corrugator supercilii (deep)

Depressor supercilii (deep)

Orbicularis oculi (superficial)

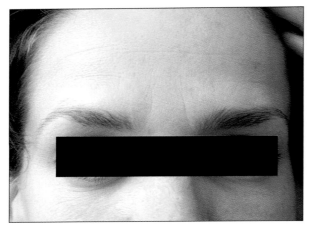

Fig. 4.2 Hyperkinetic facial lines in the upper face

clinician should also strive to learn the patient's motivation for treatment and their expectations with respect to outcome. Regardless of whether the clinician deems the procedure to have been successful, a patient who approaches BTX-A treatment with unrealistic assumptions is unlikely to be satisfied with the outcome. Much can be learned in this regard by taking a careful history of prior cosmetic interventions and the patient's degree of satisfaction with the results.

Documentation

Photographic documentation should be undertaken before and after the procedure, and particular attention should be paid to atypical facial features. While conventional film photography was commonly used in the past, digital photography offers several advantages. First, it provides superior archiving and reproduction of stored images. Second, many digital cameras will provide the option to capture video as well as still images. Video is particularly valuable in demonstrating the dynamic effects of BTX-A treatment.

Treatment of the Upper Face

Cosmetic use of BTX-A began in the upper face with treatment of glabellar lines and, to date, the upper face has yielded the greatest wealth of clinical experience with BTX-A.

Glabellar frown lines, horizontal forehead lines, and crow's feet are common presentations in the

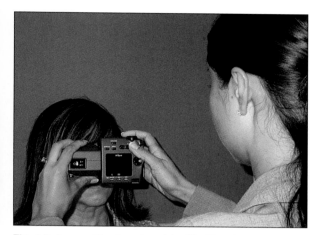

Fig. 4.3 Areas of treatment are identified by photographing the face at rest and during maximal facial expression

aging face. These lines and wrinkles may have a variety of causes, and in the older patient they are often due to age-related loss of dermal elasticity, which may be accelerated by photodamage, smoking, and other factors. In younger patients, however, hyperactivity of the facial muscles causes significant lines that convey an appearance of age, fatigue, and frustration. BTX-A provides a strikingly effective way to treat these facial lines by addressing the underlying muscular activity responsible for their formation. The great appeal of BTX-A lies in its ability to relax the musculature responsible for creating the lines without the need for surgical intervention.

General technique

Successful treatment depends on recognition of individual patient characteristics, and these are identified by photography of the target region both when muscles are at rest and during maximal contraction (Fig. 4.3). Precise delineation of natural muscle movement and corresponding facial rhytides may be achieved by marking the area to be injected while the patient is seated upright. Ask the patient to perform a range of facial expressions, including smiling and frowning maximally. Marking the skin to identify hyperkinetic lines (Fig. 4.4) using a soft eyeliner pencil is a valuable exercise and is particularly useful for clinicians less experienced with BTX-A.

The desired dose of BTX-A is drawn into the syringe. We use the Becton-Dickinson Ultra-Fine II short needle 0.3 mL insulin syringe. This syringe has

an integrated 30 gauge, silicon-coated needle that minimizes both pain on injection and drug waste compared to syringes with a needle hub. The needle remains sharp for approximately six cutaneous punctures, after which it should be discarded. Carefully remove the rubber stopper from the vial using a bottle opener prior to drawing up the solution. This will prevent the needle from becoming prematurely dull by being forced through the rubber stopper which can be replaced and the vial stored in the refrigerator. We have found that reconstituting with preserved saline (containing 0.9% benzyl alcohol), infusing slowly with a 30 gauge needle, and injecting small volumes of relatively concentrated solution will help to minimize pain associated with injections. Standard procedures should be followed with regard to sterility and skin preparation.

Injected local anesthesia is neither necessary nor recommended. Some patients may wish to minimize pain associated with dermal puncture and, if brief application of ice is ineffective, the use of topical local anesthetics such as LMX4, Betacaine, or EMLA can be beneficial by providing superficial anesthesia. If topical anesthetics are used, they should be applied at least 30 minutes before injection. If alcohol is applied to the injection site, it must be allowed to dry completely before commencing with injection because of toxin lability.

Injection technique is site-specific, and our injection techniques are discussed in the individual treatment sections below. It is important that the toxin be injected intramuscularly where feasible. Injections that are too shallow, where the toxin is delivered intradermally, will yield less satisfactory results although we do intentionally inject intradermally or just subdermally in some areas, for example to reduce bruising in the area of the supraorbital vessels. An effect will be noted following intradermal injection of BTX-A, but this is the result of diffusion of the toxin into the muscle fibers and will not produce the effects that result from intramuscular injection of the toxin. Injection sites are chosen to target the muscle responsible for facial expression, and are typically located in the mass of the target muscle, rather than at the exact site of maximal dermal depression. When injecting larger facial muscles, it is most efficacious to inject the toxin directly into the belly of the muscle. Diffusion through the body of a muscle will often accomplish the desired weakening of the muscle; however, multiple injection sites may be necessary, especially in

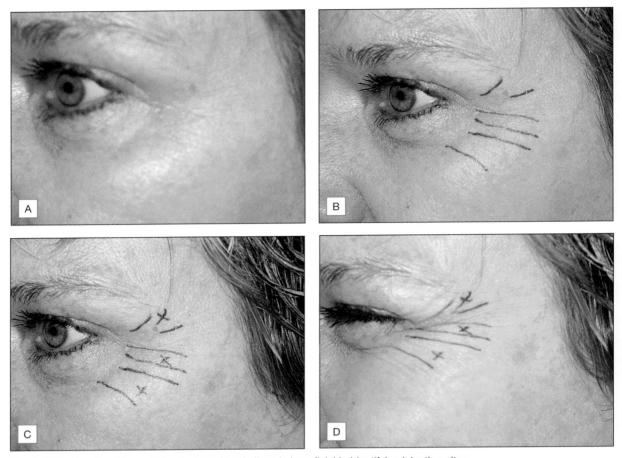

Fig. 4.4 Marking the skin to delineate hyperkinetic lines is beneficial in identifying injection sites

corrugator and orbicularis oculi where diffusion appears to be less clinically than, for example, in frontalis.

BTX and change in resting muscle tone

BTX is a neuroparalytic agent that blocks neuromuscular transmission. This produces weakness of the treated muscles. We are familiar with this effect of BTX and have used it to achieve many of its positive beneficial results. However, we are now beginning to realize that BTX produces its effects both by reduction in resting tone and also by *increasing* tone in adjacent muscles. For example, as shown in the section on brow elevation below, the brow lift we see following BTX treatment of the glabella is due to partial weakening of the glabella complex/lower frontalis producing an increase in resting tone in the untreated part of frontalis. This

complementary decrease and increase in resting tone must be borne in mind when reading the following and other chapters in this book.

Glabellar frown lines

Physical characteristics such as the type of brow arch, brow asymmetry, whether the brow is ptotic or crosses the orbital rim, and the amount of regional muscle mass may vary considerably from one individual to the next, and these factors are important in identifying appropriate doses and injection sites (Fig. 4.5). Males typically have a greater muscle mass in the brow than females, and consequently require higher doses to achieve the desired effect. Doses of 60–80 units BTX-A are often necessary to produce a reduction in glabellar lines in males, while doses of 30 or 40 units are usually sufficient to produce a satisfactory response

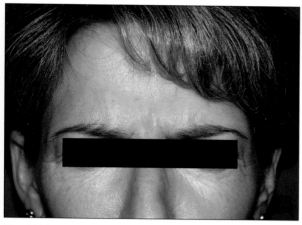

Fig. 4.5 Brow arch, asymmetry, and muscle mass are factors used in identifying injection sites

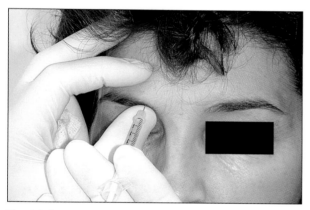

Fig. 4.6 The initial injection for glabellar frown lines is performed above the bony supraorbital ridge

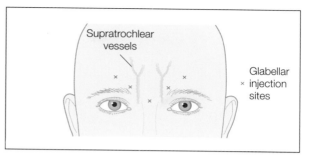

Fig. 4.7 The supratrochlear vessels are immediately medial to the injection site for glabellar frown lines

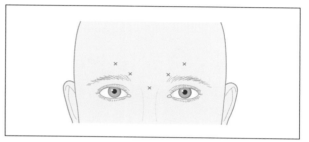

Fig. 4.8 Approximate injection sites for treatment of glabellar frown lines

in females. We have found that halving the volume of saline used to reconstitute the product provides an effective way to reduce the injected volume while doubling the dose, and this is our practice when treating males. We use an initial dose of approximately 30 and 60 units for women and men, respectively, diluted to 1 units/0.01 mL. If this does not produce the desired response, the dose is then titrated to 40 and 80 units in women and men, respectively.

The patient should be seated with the chin down and the head slightly lower than the clinician's. The needle is inserted just above the eyebrow, directly above the caruncle at the inner canthus. Regardless of eyebrow position, the injection site is always above the bony supraorbital ridge (Fig. 4.6). The supratrochlear vessels are located immediately medial to the injection site (Fig. 4.7) and it is not uncommon for some bleeding to occur, although this is rarely dramatic. It is therefore important to select a site where postinjection pressure can safely be applied.

After injecting 4–6 units, the needle is slowly withdrawn (with its tip kept superficially beneath the skin), repositioned, and advanced superiorly and superficially to at least 1 cm above the previous injection site in the orbicularis oculi. An additional 4–5 units of toxin are injected in this site. The procedure is repeated on the opposite side of the brow to ensure that a balanced appearance is maintained. A further 5–10 units are then injected into the procerus in the midline, at a point below a line joining the brows and above the crossing point of the 'X' formed by joining the medial eyebrow to the contralateral inner canthus (Fig. 4.8). In patients with horizontal brows, we inject an additional 4–5 units into a point 1 cm above the supraorbital rim in the midpupillary line (Fig. 4.9).

We instruct subjects to remain vertical for 2–3 hours following treatment. During this time, while the toxin is binding, they are instructed to frown as

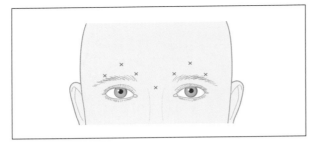

Fig. 4.9 Additional toxin is injected in patients with horizontal brows

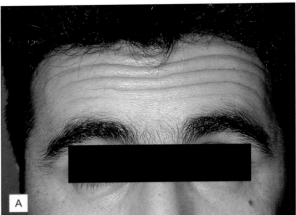

A

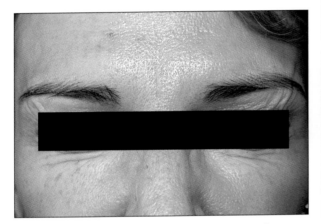

Fig. 4.10 Dramatic effects are produced by repeated treatment of glabellar frown lines

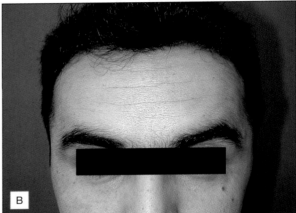

B

Fig. 4.11 Excessive weakening of the frontalis produces a lowered brow and an angry expression

much as possible, and warned not to press or otherwise manipulate the treated area. A follow-up examination should be scheduled 2–3 weeks following the initial treatment. At this time, 'touch-up' injections are performed if necessary. In patients with persistent deep resting furrows at follow-up, filling agents may be considered, although for the deeper furrows, simultaneous injection of filler will support the dermis and give an immediate enhancement of the esthetic benefit. Continued BTX-A treatment at 3- to 4-month intervals over a period of 1 year will maintain muscle weakness and produce a dramatic and lasting effect in patients with deep glabellar frown lines (Fig. 4.10). In the majority of patients, clinical benefits of BTX-A treatment for glabellar rhytides persist from 3–4 months, although in some the clinical effect may endure for 6–8 months or longer.

Horizontal forehead lines

BTX-A is effective in diminishing the appearance of undesirable horizontal forehead lines, and the effects typically last for 4–6 months. However, treatment of horizontal forehead lines requires a cautious approach. Excessive weakening of the frontalis muscle in the absence of a corresponding weakening of the depressors will result in unopposed action of the depressors, yielding a lowered brow and an angry, aggressive expression (Fig. 4.11). A conservative approach to injecting the forehead will ensure that sufficient function remains intact to avoid this unwanted outcome. Injection sites must be kept well above the brow to avoid brow ptosis as well as loss of expressivity (Fig. 4.12). Patients with a narrow brow (defined as less than 12 cm between the temporal fusion lines at midbrow level) are treated with fewer injections (four sites, compared to five) and lower doses than individuals with broader brows.

In our experience, in females a total of 48 units injected half into the elevator (frontalis) and half

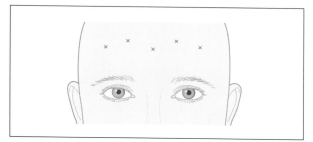

Fig. 4.12 Injection sites for horizontal forehead lines must be kept well above the brow

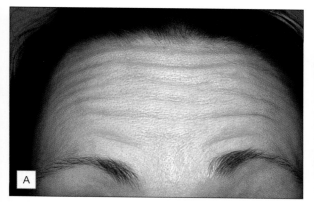

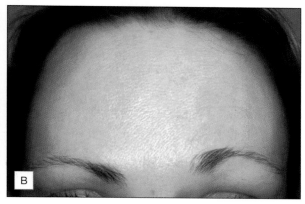

Fig. 4.13 BTX-A treatment produces dramatic improvement in horizontal forehead lines

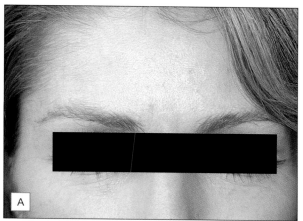

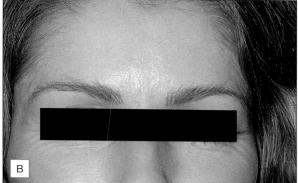

Fig. 4.14 Lateral and mid-pupil elevation following BTX-A injection in the glabellar region

into the depressors (procerus and lateral orbicularis oculi) produces maximum improvement in horizontal forehead lines and a satisfactory duration of response (Fig. 4.13). It is important to remember, however, that adverse effects are dose-related.

Brow shaping

BTX-A injections in the glabellar region can be used to alter the shape of the eyebrows to produce a more esthetically pleasing appearance. This requires a thorough understanding of the action of BTX-A in the glabellar region.

Brow elevation

Several reports have described the elevation of the brow following BTX-A treatment of glabellar lines, and we have demonstrated the beneficial result of lateral and mid-pupil elevation following injection of 20–40 units BTX-A in the glabellar region alone (Fig. 4.14). At first we believed that this was due to the action of the toxin on the medial depressors (corrugator supercilii, procerus, and the medial portion of the orbicularis oculi). We subsequently performed a small study that demonstrated that BTX-A treatment of the depressors alone (medial and lateral) would produce brow elevation and this has been confirmed by other authors.

However, a more rigorous analysis of brow height following glabella injection alone had interesting results. A total of 10 units BTX-A injected in the glabella produced mild, medial brow ptosis that persisted for 2 months. Injections of 20–40 units produced an initial lateral eyebrow elevation, followed by central and medial eyebrow elevation that peaked at 12 weeks but was still significantly present at 16 weeks. Peak effect typically occurs in skeletal muscle at 4 weeks, and this observation marks our first experience of peak effect occurring at 12 weeks. Based on the finding that the primary effect is lateral, an area not injected, we now believe that the brow lift is caused by partial inactivation of the frontalis and not by the action on the brow depressors. It is possible that a gradual lift follows the adjustment of resting tone in the frontalis muscle, causing an elevation of the central and medial eyebrow. In other words, the elevation of the eyebrows is due to an increase in tone in the untreated part of frontalis, which in turn is due to the reduction in tone in the treated part of frontalis.

The implication of this new understanding is that it is adjustment in the amount of treated frontalis that is the main factor in determining change in eyebrow position and shape. Reducing the amount of treated frontalis (for example by reducing the dose) will decrease the brow elevation and, in an extreme instance, can actually cause brow ptosis, as shown above. Similarly, moving the treated area of frontalis medially or laterally can affect eyebrow shape. This can be a very individual response and it is important that very accurate records are kept to show exact injection patterns so that these can be changed based on the initial response to treatment.

Eyebrow asymmetry

BTX-A injections provide a nonsurgical means to produce greater symmetry of the eyebrows. In general, the aim of treatment is to elevate the lower eyebrow to the same level as the higher. This can be achieved both by reducing depressor activity and by increasing tone in relevant parts of frontalis, as described above. However, in some cases part of an eyebrow may be extremely elevated and it is therefore appropriate to drop that part at the same time as the other eyebrow is being elevated in order to achieve symmetry (Fig. 4.15).

Other authors have described a technique in the glabella area whereby injection deeply into corrugator above the inner canthus will tend to preferentially affect the depressor muscles and produce

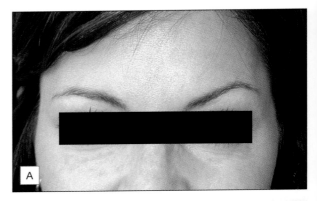

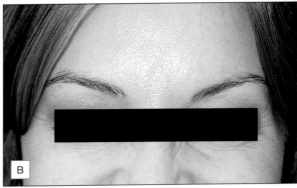

Fig. 4.15 Eyebrow asymmetry can be effectively corrected with BTX-A treatment

more brow elevation, whereas more superficial injection will have a greater effect on the inferomedial portion of frontalis and therefore cause less central brow elevation. We have two concerns about this technique. First, BTX diffuses extremely well and we have not seen differences in injection site of a few millimeters make a dramatic difference in the end result. Second, as we have shown above, we believe that the BTX brow lift is due to BTX treatment of frontalis causing an increased tone in the untreated part of frontalis. Therefore, it could be argued that the above technique could have quite the opposite effect. So far, sufficient evidence does not exist to support either position.

Assessment of the individual both at rest and dynamically, before and after treatment, is extremely important, and accurate recording of injection pattern and dose is vital to maintaining successful correction. Eyebrow asymmetry is common in all individuals and may be relatively unnoticeable. However, minor degrees of asymmetry occurring after brow lift surgery can cause great anguish to both patient and physician. Fortunately BTX-A

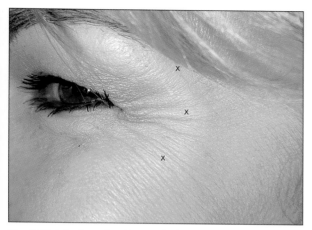

Fig. 4.16 Injection sites for crow's feet are identified while the patient is smiling maximally

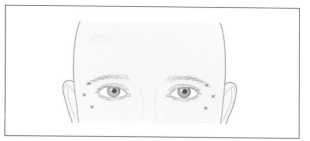

Fig. 4.17 Approximate injection sites for treatment of crow's feet

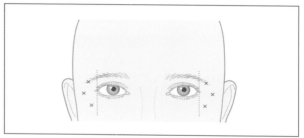

Fig. 4.18 Regardless of distribution of crow's feet, the most anterior injection should be placed lateral to a line drawn vertically from the lateral canthus

offers a simple way of correcting this in the post-surgical patient.

Crow's feet

BTX-A can dramatically reduce the appearance of crow's feet rhytides by relaxing or weakening (as opposed to paralyzing) the lateral orbicularis oculi, and this treatment is effective even in patients with severely photodamaged skin. Typically, two to three injection sites lateral to the lateral orbital rim are used, and equal doses of toxin (approximately 4–7 units/site; 12–20 units/side) are injected into each site. Reports detailing optimal dosage in the lateral orbital region vary. One recent dose-ranging study found no significant difference in efficacy between 6 units/side and 18 units/side. Other reported total dose ranges include 5–15 units and 4–5 units per eye over two or three injection sites. We inject 12–15 units/side, distributed equally over two to four sites. To minimize bruising, we recommend using as few and as superficial injections as possible.

Injection sites for crow's feet are determined while the patient is smiling maximally (Fig. 4.16). Identify the center of the crow's feet. The first injection site is in the center of the area of maximal wrinkling, approximately 1–2 cm lateral to the lateral orbital rim. The second and third injection sites are approximately 1–1.5 cm above and below the first injection site, respectively (Fig. 4.17). In some patients, crow's feet are distributed equally above and below the lateral canthus; in others, crow's feet exist primarily below the lateral canthus. In the latter case, the injection sites may be in a line that angles from anteroinferior to superoposterior. In all patients, regardless of distribution of crow's feet, the most anterior injection should be placed lateral to a line drawn vertically from the lateral canthus (Fig. 4.18). It is important that the injections be performed when the patient is not smiling. If the patient is smiling, the toxin may affect the ipsilateral zygomaticus complex, causing ptosis of the upper lip. Clinical effects from the first injection session typically persist for approximately 4 months. However, following subsequent treatments, the effects may last for more than 4 months (Fig. 4.19).

Effects

Clinical effects

The clinical effects of BTX-A typically appear 1–4 days following treatment. Peak effect is seen at 1–4 weeks, with a gradual decline after 3–4 months. The literature indicates a fairly consistent onset of effect, although the duration of effect has been reported to vary. Extended duration of effect, lasting from 6 months to a year, has been observed

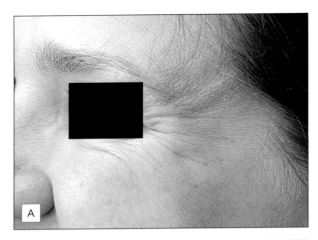

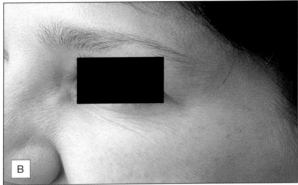

Fig. 4.19 Patient before and after BTX-A treatment for crow's feet

safe, and there have been no reports of long-term adverse effects or health hazards associated with any cosmetic indication for BTX-A.

In a recent review of 50 individuals treated with BTX-A for cosmetic purposes for at least 5 years and with at least 10 treatment sessions each, there was a minimal incidence (less than 1%) of mild and transient eyelid or eyebrow ptosis. There were no serious long-term adverse events.

Brow ptosis

The most serious complications of BTX-A treatment in the upper face are brow and eyelid ptosis and asymmetrical changes to the appearance of the eyebrows. Brow ptosis is the result of poor injection technique during glabellar or brow treatment and occurs when the injected toxin affects too much frontalis. We believe a higher concentration of toxin enables more accurate placement, greater duration of effect, and fewer side effects. Lower concentrations encourage the spread of toxin, as there is a radius of denervation associated with each point of injection due to toxin spread of about 1–1.5 cm (diameter 2–3 cm). The patient must be instructed to remain upright, to avoid rubbing or manipulating the injected area for 2 hours, and to exercise the treated muscles as much as possible during the first 4 hours following treatment.

Brow ptosis most commonly occurs after injection of frontalis, particularly to treat horizontal forehead lines. It produces an extremely negative appearance and can persist for up to 3 months. Appropriate patient selection (especially avoiding injecting frontalis in individuals with significant brow ptosis) and pre-injection of the brow depressors if necessary (i.e. in patients with low-set brows or mild brow ptosis, and those over the age of 50 years) will help avoid this outcome. It is our practice to *always* inject the depressors when we are treating frontalis, even in younger individuals.

To minimize the diminished expressiveness that may occur following injection of the frontalis lateral to the mid-pupillary line, inject above the lowest fold produced when the patient elevates the frontalis and limit the treatment of forehead lines to the portion 3 cm or more above the brow (Fig. 4.20). Brow ptosis is more likely to result if the glabella and the whole forehead are injected in a single session. Apraclonidine (Iopidine 0.5%), alpha-adrenergic agonist ophthalmic eye drops that stimulate Müller's

in patients treated repeatedly over the course of a year or more. Our experience corroborates this observation, and it appears that the duration of clinical effect may be related to the total number of treatment sessions. This also suggests that BTX-A has a clinical effect that persists beyond the duration of the direct effect of the drug on muscle activity.

Adverse effects and complications

The safety of BTX-A treatment is well established. Adverse effects are usually mild and transient and are associated with poor injection technique and/or inappropriate patient selection. Transient adverse events include swelling or bruising at the injection site, mild headache, and flu-like symptoms. It has been observed that smaller doses are less likely to cause problems than larger doses, and for this reason a conservative approach is recommended in most patients. On the whole, the treatment is extremely

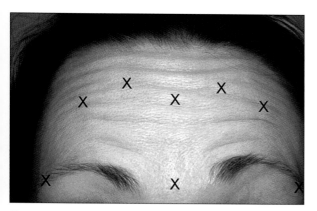

Fig. 4.20 When treating the frontalis, inject above the lowest fold produced when the patient elevates the frontalis and limit injections to the portion 3 cm or more above the brow

muscle, can be used to disguise mild brow ptosis, though it should be noted that allergic contact conjunctivitis can occur with the prolonged use of apraclonidine.

Upper eyelid ptosis

Upper eyelid ptosis occurs when the toxin diffuses through the orbital septum, affecting the upper eyelid levator muscle (Fig. 4.21). This complication is most commonly seen following treatment of the glabellar complex, and as with brow ptosis, is the result of poor injection technique. Ptosis may be evident as early as 48 hours or as late as 14 days after injection and may last from 2 to 12 weeks. To minimize the possibility of eyelid ptosis, avoid large injection volumes, accurately place injections no closer than 1 cm above the central bony orbital rim,

and advise patients to remain upright and not to manipulate the injected area for several hours after injection. Do not inject at or under the mid-brow. Apraclonidine 0.5% eye drops can be used in eyelid ptosis. It will lift the lid by 1–2 mm and compensate for the weakness of the levator palpebrae superioris by stimulating contraction of an adrenergic muscle, Müller's muscle, which is located immediately below the levator muscle. One or two drops three times a day can be continued until the ptosis resolves.

Cocked eyebrow

Inappropriate injection of the medial fibers of the frontalis muscle can cause the untreated lateral fibers of the frontalis to pull upward on the brow, producing a quizzical or 'cockeyed' appearance (Fig. 4.22). This can be corrected by injecting 2–3 units of BTX-A into the fibers of the lateral forehead

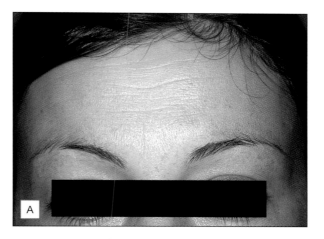

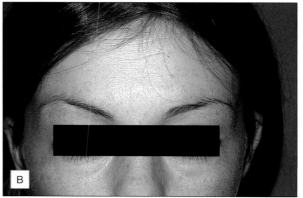

Fig. 4.22 Inappropriate injection of the medial fibers of the frontalis muscle can produce a cockeyed appearance

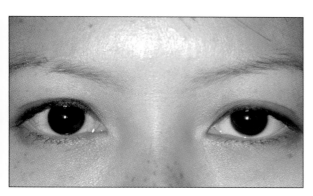

Fig. 4.21 Upper eyelid ptosis

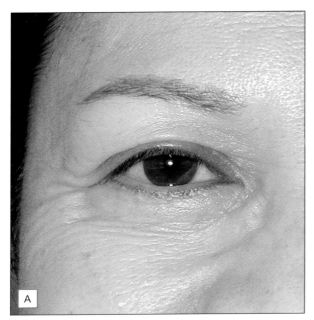 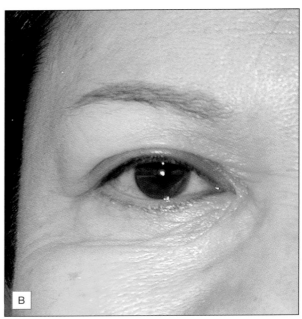

Fig. 4.23 A drooping lateral lower eyelid may occur following periorbital BTX-A treatment

which are exerting the upward pull. Only a small amount of BTX-A is required, and a cautious approach is necessary, as overcompensation can yield an irreversible and unsightly hooded brow that partially covers the eye. Avoidance of this complication with future BTX-A treatments is by keeping the glabellar treatments more medial so that the increased tone in frontalis produces a smooth arch to the brow rather than the 'Jack Nicholson' or 'Spock' look.

Periorbital complications

Periorbital complications following BTX-A treatment include bruising, diplopia, ectropion, or a drooping lateral lower eyelid (Fig. 4.23). An asymmetrical smile may result if the toxin spreads to the zygomaticus major (Fig. 4.24). To avoid these outcomes, inject laterally at least 1 cm outside the bony orbit, or 1.5 cm lateral to the lateral canthus, and do not inject close to the inferior margin of the zygoma. Ecchymosis can be reduced by injecting superficially in a wheal or a series of continuous blebs. Placing each injection at the advancing border of the previous injection will facilitate avoidance of blood vessels. In some individuals, asking them to perform a Valsalva maneuver immediately before injection will display blood vessels that may otherwise have been hidden under the skin.

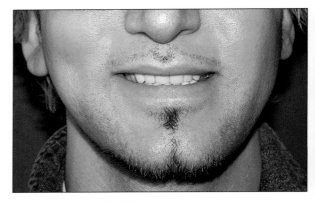

Fig. 4.24 Spread of BTX-A to the zygomaticus major may cause an asymmetrical smile. Note slight left upper lip droop

Conclusion

BTX-A is safe and effective as primary therapy for correction of dynamic facial lines caused by underlying muscle activity. Clinicians with a sound understanding of facial anatomy can use BTX-A to dramatic effect in appropriately selected individuals. Complications and adverse outcomes can be minimized, and the clinical benefits of the treatment maximized, by developing good injection technique and using the lowest effective dose. The increasing use of BTX-A in the practice of cosmetic dermatology is a reflection of its striking benefits across a broad range of indications. BTX-A does not replace surgery, skin resurfacing, or soft-tissue augmentation, but it represents an extremely valuable part of the clinical armamentarium, one whose utility and practical applications will continue to expand. BTX-A is a powerful treatment adjunct as well as a unique and positive esthetic primary treatment.

Further Reading

Ahn MS, Catten M, Maas CS 2000 Temporal brow lift using botulinum toxin A. Plastic and Reconstructive Surgery 105:1129–1135

Carruthers A, Carruthers J 2003 Glabella BTX-A injection and eyebrow height: a further photographic analysis. Presented at the Annual Meeting of the American Academy of Dermatology, 21–26 March, San Francisco, CA

Carruthers A, Carruthers J, Cohen J 2003 A prospective, double-blind, randomized, parallel-group, dose-ranging study of botulinum toxin type a in female subjects with horizontal forehead rhytides. Dermatologic Surgery 29:461–467

Carruthers A, Carruthers J, Said S 2001 Dose-ranging study of botulinum toxin type A in the treatment of glabellar lines. Poster presentation, American Academy of Dermatology Annual Meeting.

Carruthers J, Carruthers A 2001 BOTOX use in the mid and lower face and neck. Seminars in Cutaneous Medicine and Surgery 20:85–92

Carruthers J, Carruthers A 2003 A prospective, randomized, parallel group study analyzing the effect of BTX-A (BOTOX) and nonanimal sourced hyaluronic acid (NASHA, Restylane) in combination compared with NASHA (Restylane) alone in severe glabellar rhytides in adult female subjects: treatment of severe glabellar rhytides with a hyaluronic acid derivative compared with the derivative and BTX-A. Dermatologic Surgery 29:802–809

Carruthers J, Weiss RW, Narurkar V, Flynn TC 2003 Intense pulsed light and botulinum toxin type A for the aging face. Cosmetic Dermatology 16:2–16

Carruthers JA, Lowe NJ, Menter MA, et al 2002 A multicentre, double-blind, randomized, placebo-controlled study of efficacy and safety of botulinum toxin type A in the treatment of glabellar lines. Journal of the American Academy of Dermatology 46: 840–849

Carruthers JDA and Carruthers JA 1992 Treatment of glabellar frown lines with C. botulinum-A exotoxin. Journal of Dermatologic Surgery and Oncology 18:17-21

Fagien S, Brandt FS 2001 Primary and adjunctive use of botulinum toxin type A (Botox) in facial aesthetic surgery: beyond the glabella. Clinics in Plastic Surgery 28:127–148

Flynn TC, Carruthers A, Carruthers J 2002 Surgical pearl: the use of the Ultra-Fine II short needle 0.3-cc insulin syringe for botulinum toxin injections. Journal of the American Academy of Dermatology 46:931–933

Garcia A, Fulton JE Jr 1996 Cosmetic denervation of the muscles of facial expression with botulinum toxin: a dose–response study. Dermatologic Surgery 22:39–43

Hexsel DM, Trindade de Almeida A, Rutowitsch M, et al 2003 Multicenter, double-blind study of the efficacy of injections with botulinum toxin type A reconstituted up to six consecutive weeks before application. Dermatologic Surgery 29:523–529

Huang W, Rogachefsky AS, Foster JA 2000 Brow lift with botulinum toxin. Dermatologic Surgery 26:55–60

Huilgol SC, Carruthers A, Carruthers JDA 2000 Raising eyebrows with botulinum toxin. Dermatologic Surgery 25:373–376

Keen M, Kopelman JE, Aviv JE, et al 1994 Botulinum toxin: a novel method to remove periorbital wrinkles. Facial Plastic Surgery 10: 141–146

Klein AW 1998 Dilution and storage of botulinum toxin. Dermatologic Surgery 24:1179–1180

Klein AW 2003 Complications, adverse reactions, and insights with the use of botulinum toxin. Dermatological Surgery 29: 549–556

Lowe NJ, Lask G, Yamauchi P, et al 2002 Bilateral, double-blind, randomized comparison of three doses of botulinum toxin type A and placebo in patients with crow's feet. Journal of the American Academy of Dermatology 47:834–840

5

Periocular Treatment

Brian Biesman, Kenneth A. Arndt

Introduction

Esthetic rejuvenation of the periocular region is a common goal shared by millions of people today. While some individuals present with specific complaints about eyelid position, lateral canthal (crow's feet) rhytids or eyebrow position, many others simply complain of looking tired or sad when they feel well. Treatment of these patients requires a comprehensive knowledge of the involutional changes that commonly occur in the periorbital region, the underlying bony and soft-tissue anatomy, the relationship of the eye to the orbital rim, and, of course, the person's expectations.

It is most helpful to begin this discussion reviewing pertinent periorbital anatomic structures and their functional correlation to ocular and facial esthetics. Eyelid skin is amongst the thinnest in the body with little dermal collagen. It is dynamic, moves frequently with blinking, and is located in an anatomic region that receives extensive exposure to sunlight. It is therefore no surprise that eyelid and periocular skin is highly prone to actinic injury with thinning, loss of elasticity, dyspigmentation, and the development of fine wrinkling.

Downward movement of the eyebrows is another common occurrence with aging. Eyebrow ptosis may present as 'hooding' of the upper eyelids, horizontal forehead rhytids from chronic brow elevation, horizontal rhytids at the nasion, and even headache and fatigue. Brow ptosis develops insidiously and many affected patients fail to recognize this change themselves. A history of 'looking better' when a towel has been wrapped around the head after showering is highly suggestive of brow ptosis. Significant brow ptosis can also accentuate superiorly located lateral canthal crow's feet lines. Failure to recognize brow ptosis can have disastrous consequences if botulinum toxin (BTX) injections are administered in an effort to treat horizontal fore-head rhytids. In this scenario, relaxation of the frontalis muscle will prevent elevation of the brows leaving an uncompensated ptosis (and a *de*compensated patient!). This is referred to as latent brow ptosis and can be identified by manually holding the brows in a fixed position as the patient gazes straight ahead. Brow configuration varies widely from patient to patient. In many cases it is impossible to determine whether the brows have actually fallen or whether they were always low. When asked, most patients are uncertain whether their brow position has changed. The best way to evaluate this is to examine old photographs. It is most instructive to study at least one photo per decade starting in the teenage years (e.g. High School yearbook). Reposi-tioning of brows via surgical or chemical techniques can be highly rewarding but can also change a patient's fundamental appearance. This must be carefully discussed prior to treatment.

Eyelid position relative to the eye itself must also be carefully assessed. The eyelids should be studied both at rest and while animating. Normally the upper eyelid margin covers the superior 1–2 mm of the cornea while the lower eyelid margin rests at the corneoscleral limbus. The white colored sclera should not be visible at either the 06:00 or 12:00 positions. The distance between the edge of the upper and lower eyelids while the patient gazes straight ahead in primary position is referred to as the palpebral fissure or palpebral aperture. While ethnic and interpatient variations exist, the normal palpebral fissure measures 8–11 mm (Fig. 5.1) The palpebral fissure normally narrows with smiling. Failure of this subtle change to occur with facial animation may be interpreted by others as unnatural or insincere. Upper eyelid position is usually judged relative to the pupil or superior limbus. There is a wide range of 'normal', with some patients having naturally low upper lids while others have a wide

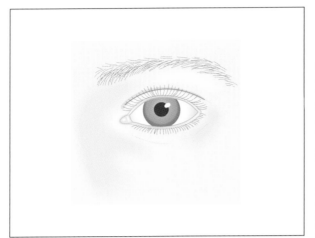

Fig. 5.1 Normal upper and lower eyelid position relative to the eye. (Adapted from Fig. 20.2, Biesman BS, Iwamoto M 2002 Blepharoplasty. In: Kaminer MS, Dover JS, Arndt KA (eds) Atlas of Cosmetic Surgery. WB Saunders, Philadelphia)

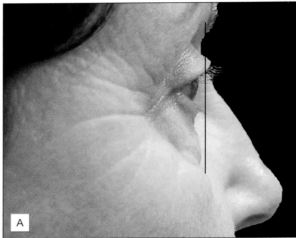

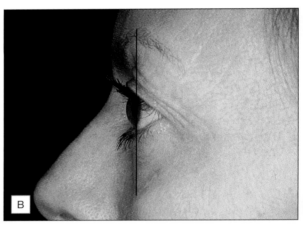

Fig. 5.2 (**A**) A vertical plane parallel to the anterior surface of the malar eminence passes anterior to the cornea. There is good bony support for this eyelid. (**B**) A vertical plane parallel to the anterior surface of the malar eminence passes through the eye. This lid is at risk of developing ectropion following botulinum toxin injections in the pretarsal region. (Fig. 20.2, Biesman BS, Iwamoto M 2002 Blepharoplasty. In: Kaminer MS, Dover JS, Arndt KA (eds) Atlas of Cosmetic Surgery. WB Saunders, Philadelphia)

palpebral fissure. Blepharoptosis is the term used to describe a lid that is in a lower than desirable position. Ptosis is thus a relative, as opposed to an absolute, condition. A ptotic upper eyelid may occlude some, none, or even the entire pupil. Many patients are highly sensitive to changes in their upper eyelid position although most do not become aware of their eyelid position until after undergoing a periorbital procedure such as BTX injection or blepharoplasty surgery. The value of preoperative photographs and identification of pretreatment asymmetry cannot be overstated.

In a situation analogous to eyebrow ptosis, latent ptosis of the upper eyelid may be present in an individual who presents with a chief complaint of horizontal forehead rhytids. These patients chronically elevate their lids and brows to compensate for the superior visual field limitation induced by the eyelid position. In this setting, injection of BTX into the frontalis muscle will uncover the previously compensated ptosis. As with latent brow ptosis, latent eyelid ptosis can be detected by manually fixating the brows in a relaxed position and examining the patient as they gaze straight ahead.

The lower eyelid serves two major functions: protection of the eye and direction of tears toward the lacrimal punctae located in the extreme medial portion of the eyelid margin. The normal lower eyelid has a gentle upsweep laterally such that the lateral canthal angle is 2 mm higher than that of the medial canthus. Lower eyelid position is also

somewhat dependent on the position of the eye relative to the orbital rim. This can be determined by drawing a plane parallel to the face through the anterior-most projection of the cornea. When viewed sagitally, if this plane passes through the lower eyelid or cheek, there is good bony support for the eyelid. If, however, the plane passes anterior to the malar eminence, there is relatively little eyelid support and these patients are much more prone to ectropion development following surgery or BTX injection (Figs 5.2A and 5.2B). Lower eyelid position is also determined in part by the relative

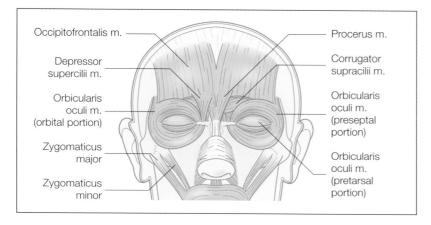

Occipitofrontalis m.

Depressor
supercilii m.

Orbicularis
oculi m.
(orbital portion)

Zygomaticus
major

Zygomaticus
minor

Procerus m.

Corrugator
supracilii m.

Orbicularis
oculi m.
(preseptal
portion)

Orbicularis
oculi m.
(pretarsal
portion)

Fig. 5.3 Anatomy of orbicularis oculi
muscle and related structures

integrity of the medial and lateral canthal tendons (see below). Canthal tendon laxity occurs normally with aging. In the setting of mild to moderate laxity, lids may maintain normal position and function, especially if adequate bony support is present. With increasing laxity, the lid will sag visibly, exposing the sclera below the inferior corneoscleral limbus. This condition is referred to as ectropion. Many patients have enough residual canthal tendon tone that the lower eyelid position remains acceptable from functional and esthetic standpoints, but do not have enough integrity to avoid ectropion formation when additional stresses such as BTX injections or surgery are introduced. Lower eyelid integrity may be assessed with the 'snap' or 'pinch' tests. The snap test is performed by pulling the lid downward and letting the lid return to its resting position. A brisk return is considered normal. A slow, gradual response is abnormal and suggestive of increased risk for ectropion formation or tearing following BTX injections. The pinch test, somewhat less popular than the snap test, is performed by pinching the lower eyelid between the thumb and forefinger and distracting it from the globe. Less than 6 mm is considered normal. If the lid stretches further than 6 mm, caution should be undertaken when performing lower eyelid procedures.

While upper eyelid position is highly variable, lower eyelid position is less so. Rounding of the lateral canthus or temporal ectropion can be interpreted as a sad or artificial look and should be avoided. Potential changes in lower eyelid position must be discussed prior to BTX injection.

Beneath the eyelid skin is found the orbicularis oculi muscle. When this muscle contracts it forcibly closes the eyelids. The orbicularis oculi muscle is divided into pretarsal, preseptal, and orbital components. The pretarsal component overlies the tarsal plates, the collagenous 'backbone' of the eyelid, while the preseptal portion overlies the orbital septum, a fibrous membrane separating the orbital contents from more superficial structures. At its medial aspect, the pretarsal orbicularis muscle fibers condense to form the medial canthal tendon (MCT), a firm structure that inserts on the medial orbital rim. Laterally, the pretarsal orbicularis fibers from the upper and lower lids join to form the lateral canthal tendon, analogous structure to the MCT that inserts inside the lateral orbital rim (Fig. 5.3). If the pretarsal orbicularis muscle is rendered inactive while the preseptal portion of the muscle is allowed to contract, the preseptal portion of the muscle can move upward in an 'overriding' fashion, turning the eyelashes and lid margin in against the globe, a condition known as entropion. Relative hypertrophy of the pretarsal orbicularis muscle produces 'bunching' of the lower eyelids that occurs with smiling. If this condition is treated with BTX, the injections should be administered into the pretarsal and superior preseptal muscle. The orbital portion of the orbicularis oculi muscle overlies the orbital rim and blends with the frontalis, procerus, depressor supercilii, and corrugator supraciliaris muscles of the eyebrow superiorly, and the temporalis and zygomaticus major and minor muscles laterally and inferiorly (Fig. 5.3). The temporal portion of the orbital orbicularis oculi muscle is the primary eyebrow depressor.

The orbital portion of the orbicularis muscle is highly variable in size and shape, especially laterally and inferiorly. Temporally the orbicularis oculi muscle fans out from the lateral canthus toward the ear. In some patients the muscle extends only as far as the outer aspect of the orbital rim while in others it extends almost to the tragus. The muscle also extends to a variable degree superiorly and inferiorly. The distribution of the orbicularis oculi muscle is assessed by asking the patient to forcibly close their eyes. Digital palpation is then used to determine the muscle's size and shape. Asymmetry of the orbicularis oculi muscle is common so the muscle should be assessed on each side prior to BTX injection. The dose and distribution pattern of the toxin is entirely dependent on the orbicularis oculi muscle size and shape. Although general guidelines can be created, the concept of a 'standard' dose and distribution pattern of BTX does not apply in the periorbital region.

The primary elevator of the upper eyelid is the levator palpebrae superioris muscle. This muscle arises from the lesser wing of the sphenoid, courses anteriorly along the orbital roof, and then develops a broad aponeurosis that splits into two leaves. The posterior leaf inserts on the tarsal plate while the anterior leaf passes through the orbicularis muscle and inserts into the skin, forming the eyelid crease. As a skeletal muscle, the levator is susceptible to weakening if exposed to BTX. The secondary elevator of the upper eyelid, formally named the superior tarsal muscle, is usually referred to as Müller's muscle. Müller's muscle lies between conjunctiva and the levator palpebrae superioris and inserts on the superior tarsal border (Fig. 5.4). In contrast to levator, Müller's muscle is an adrenergically innervated smooth muscle that is not significantly affected by the action of BTX. This difference has a useful clinical correlate in that administration of a topical adrenergic agonist can correct some or all of the ptosis that may result if the levator palpebrae superioris is inadvertently exposed to BTX.

Anatomy of Crow's Feet Lateral Orbital Rhytids

Lines emanating from the lateral canthal region in a fan-shaped distribution are commonly referred to as crow's feet lines. These lines may be caused by contraction of the orbicularis oculi muscle alone but skin laxity and contraction of zygomaticus major may contribute to varying degrees as well. Crow's feet lines are normal and may appear as early as the late teenage years. With progressive deepening or enlargement, crow's feet lines are considered to stigmatize aging or fatigue. Factors that contribute

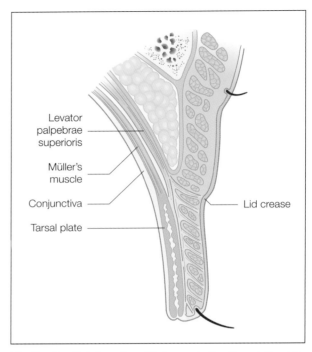

Fig. 5.4 Sagittal view of eyelid demonstrating the relationship of the upper eyelid retractors to the tarsal plate. (Fig. 20.6A, Biesman BS, Iwamoto M 2002 Blepharoplasty. In: Kaminer MS, Dover JS, Arndt KA (eds) Atlas of Cosmetic Surgery. WB Saunders, Philadelphia)

to increasing prominence of crow's feet include photoaging, amount of subcutaneous fat, general health, smoking, and prolonged contraction of the orbicularis muscle as is seen in fishermen, farmers, life guards, and others with occupational exposure to sunlight. Some patients have deep rhytids in repose while others only demonstrate deep lines with animation. It is extremely important to distinguish between lines caused by orbicularis contraction versus those produced by a 'smiling effect' as contraction of the zygomaticus muscles 'pushes' skin into the periorbital region. The latter phenomenon is difficult to treat without risking facial droop or an unnatural appearance as overtreatment of the zygomaticus muscle will decrease the natural cheek elevation and fullness that occurs with smiling (Figs 5.5A and 5.5B).

Indications for the use of BTX in the periocular region

It is critically important to understand exactly what feature of the periocular region is most objectionable before making therapeutic recommendations.

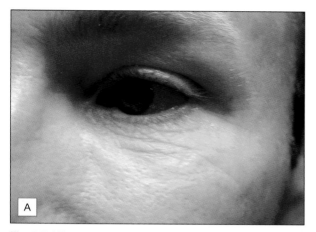 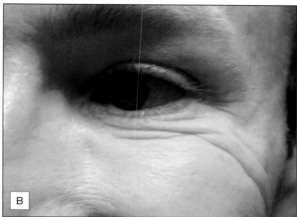

Fig. 5.5 (**A**) A 35-year-old male in repose. (**B**) Same patient, smiling. Note vertical shortening of lower eyelid and upward movement of cheek due to contraction of zygomaticus muscles

Some patients complain of 'looking tired' when in fact they are concerned about loss of skin tone, excessive eyelid skin (dermatochalasis), eyebrow ptosis, dark circles under the eyes, hollowness in the tear trough area (medial lower eyelid below the orbital rim), bulging orbital fat pads, 'hypertrophic' orbicularis oculi muscle, and/or deep lateral canthal rhytids. Periocular rejuvenation is a complex topic and addressing only one of many needs may or may not provide a satisfactory result. The best candidates for periocular BTX injections are those with mild to moderately deep lateral canthal rhytids and/or those who develop a 'roll' of pretarsal orbicularis muscle as they smile. There are very few absolute contraindications to periocular BTX injection. It should be used with great caution in:

- patients with dry eyes such as in true dry eye syndrome or systemic diseases that may produce dry eyes such as Sjögren's syndrome and severe rheumatoid arthritis
- patients with ocular myasthenia gravis or other conditions that may affect extraocular muscle function
- patients whose eyes do not close well (a condition known as lagophthalmos) due to previous 7th nerve palsy, thyroid eye disease, or blepharoplasty surgery.

Patient evaluation

Evaluation begins with a medical and surgical history, focusing special attention to prior blepharoplasty, brow, midface, or face lifting, ablative periocular resurfacing, injection of fillers, or BTX. An ophthalmic history should include questions about general ocular health but should specifically address tearing, dry eyes, and previous kerato-refractive surgery (e.g. LASIK). Patients who have undergone LASIK surgery have a high incidence of dry eye. Weakening the orbicularis oculi muscle with BTX injections may impair eyelid function to the point that dry eye symptoms may worsen. Conversely, if a patient who is used to receiving periorbital BTX injections decides to undergo LASIK surgery shortly after BTX injection, it is advisable to reduce the dose of toxin administered, to administer injections slightly further from the lateral canthus and, if lower eyelid injections are typically given, to reduce the dose or even eliminate this area altogether. The patient should then be re-evaluated after the LASIK procedure is complete. If symptoms of dry eye syndrome are absent, additional BTX injections may be administered as needed to satisfy the patient's esthetic needs. The medical history should include particular attention to disorders that can affect the eyes or tear film such as Graves' disease, Hashimoto's thyroiditis, and collagen vascular diseases.

Examination of the patient begins with evaluation of the patient literally from across the room. The patient's facial features are assessed for typical facial stigmata of aging including lentigenes, erythema, fine wrinkling, loss of skin laxity, eyebrow and/or eyelid ptosis (or chronic eyebrow elevation to correct latent brow or lid ptosis), midfacial ptosis, jowling, loss of facial volume, and deep dynamic rhytids in the glabellar, perioral, and periocular regions. It is particularly important to view the patient as a whole before concentrating on the periocular (or any other individual) region as the goal of any treatment is to create a harmonious facial appearance. The eye is drawn to asymmetry more so than rhytids or lines. That is to say, creation of a 'smooth island in a sea of rhytids' produces a less natural appearance than if the patient were not treated at all.

The patient is then evaluated from a frontal perspective. Particular attention is paid to the presence of rhytids at rest, eyebrow contour and position, horizontal forehead rhytids that may be indicative of chronic brow elevation, extent of photoaging, presence of dermatochalasis in the upper eyelid, position of the upper eyelid margin relative to the pupil, and lower eyelid position. If white sclera is visible above the superior limbus or below the inferior corneoscleral limbus, additional ophthalmic evaluation is warranted. The presence of horizontal forehead rhytids may either indicate overactive use of the muscles or facial expression or a compensatory response to eyebrow ptosis. One must make this distinction as weakening the frontalis muscle in the latter setting will uncover a previously latent eyebrow ptosis. That is to say, patients who have been elevating their eyebrows continuously in order to prevent impairment of their superior visual field will no longer be able to do so if their frontalis muscle is weakened. The examiner can identify the patient with latent brow ptosis by studying the patient when the frontalis muscle is completely relaxed (instruct the patient to relax their forehead). If the eyebrows assume a lower position when the frontalis muscle relaxes, BTX should not be injected into the forehead. These patients need eyebrow and/or eyelid surgery to correct their underlying problem. Next, the patient is asked to gently (not forcibly) close the eyes to ensure complete apposition of the upper and lower lids. Some patients who have had prior surgery, trauma, or thyroid disease may be able to forcibly close their eyes but have an incomplete blink that leaves them highly vulnerable to symptomatic dry eyes if the orbicularis oculi muscle is weakened. The patient is then instructed to forcibly close the eyes. This permits evaluation of the pretarsal orbicularis oculi muscle in its dynamic state. The appearance of a prominent 'bulge' in the pretarsal region is suggestive of 'hypertrophic' orbicularis oculi muscle. This condition must be differentiated from a 'bunched' lower eyelid occurring as a result of cheek tissue recruitment with contraction of the zygomaticus major and minor muscles. Horizontal rhytids in the lateral canthal region should be evaluated in both frontal and lateral views. The patient is viewed from each side first at rest, then with gentle eyelid closure, and finally during forced closure. This series of maneuvers permits the examiner to differentiate between fine skin wrinkles due to loss of elasticity and rhytids caused by action of the orbicularis oculi muscle. Next, a 'map' of the orbicularis oculi muscle should be constructed by asking the patient to squeeze their eyes tightly repeatedly while the examiner palpates the lateral canthal region with the tip of the index finger. The orbicularis oculi muscle may be relatively small and confined to the region overlying the lateral orbital rim or may extend nearly to the tragus laterally, into the lateral extent of the temporal region superiorly, and into the upper region of the midface inferiorly. It is important to map the orbicularis oculi muscle on both sides as its distribution may be asymmetric. Finally, the position of the eye is assessed relative to the orbital rim. Patients with prominent eyes due to high myopia (a condition in which the globe is actually longer than normal), thyroid eye disease, or shallow orbits should be treated with greater care as they are more prone to lagophthalmos and change in lower eyelid position after BTX injection.

Treatment goals

BTX may be used in the periorbital region to diminish dynamic rhytids in the lateral canthal region, to weaken eyebrow depressors and thereby elevate or contour the brows, and to treat 'hypertrophic' orbicularis oculi muscle in the lower eyelid. In any given patient it may be desirable to accomplish one or more of these goals; they are not mutually exclusive and should be considered independently.

Lateral canthal region

When treating lateral canthal rhytids, the injector must distinguish between those lines due to the action of the orbicularis oculi muscle, those caused by contraction of zygomaticus major and minor muscles (causing upward movement of the cheek with smiling), and those due to photoaging of the skin. Only those lines clearly caused by contraction of the orbicularis oculi muscle should be treated with BTX (Figs 5.6A–D). Attempts to treat too far inferiorly may produce an unnatural appearance when smiling, facial asymmetry or, in the most extreme circumstance, facial drooping due to involvement of the zygomaticus complex. It is usually best to use the least amount of toxin necessary to produce the desired clinical effect while still providing adequate efficacy. Use of too much toxin will minimize the action of the orbicularis oculi muscle to the point where the lateral canthus does not wrinkle at all with smiling and other facial expression. This can signal insincerity and, thus, overaggressive injection in the crow's feet region should be avoided. A careful injection record should be kept (Fig. 5.7) and patients followed up 2 weeks after their injection. At the follow-up visit, the treatment goals should be reviewed and compared to the clinical results. If additional injections are needed to achieve the desired goals, these should be administered at the 2-week visit. If the patient has not achieved the best possible outcome, careful notes should be made about adjustments that need to be made in dosage, placement, or both.

Pretarsal orbicularis

BTX can also be used to weaken the pretarsal orbicularis oculi muscle. This can reduce the prominent 'roll' that appears with smiling in patients with 'hypertrophic' orbicularis muscle and can also increase the size of the palpebral fissure (the distance between the upper and lower eyelids). While these goals are separate, they are indistinct in that it is difficult to accomplish one objective without the other. That is to say, treatment of hypertrophic orbicularis oculi muscle will not only reduce the

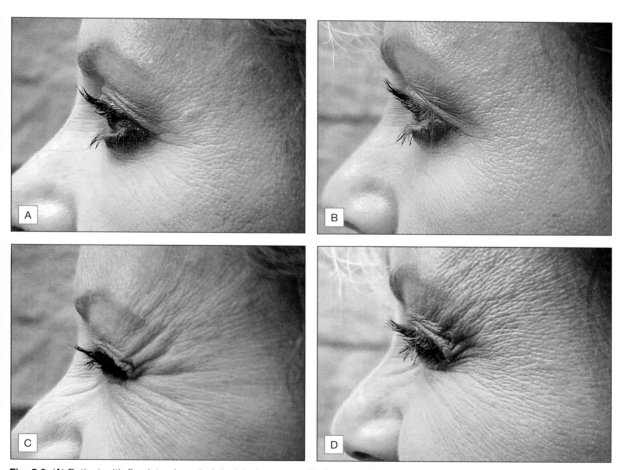

Fig. 5.6 (**A**) Patient with fine lateral canthal rhytids, in repose. (**B**) Same patient 3 weeks after injection of 10 units of BTX-A in the lateral canthal rhytids, in repose. (**C**) Same patient prior to injection demonstrating active contraction of orbicularis oculi muscle. (**D**) After BTX-A injection with active contraction of orbicularis oculi muscle

Botox Flow Sheet				
Patient name				
Date				
Concentration (units per 0.1)				
Glabella				
Forehead				
Periorbital				
Perioral				
Lateral forehead				
Neck, axilla, palms				
Total no. mL				
Total no. units				
Date mixed				
Lot no.				
Exp. date				

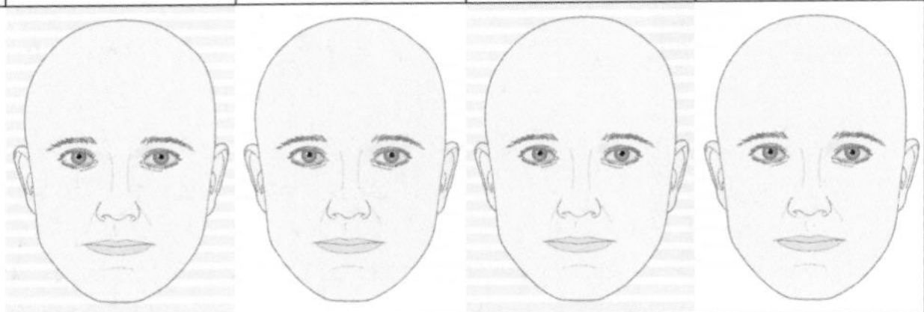

Fig. 5.7 Botox flow sheet

muscle bulk upon smiling but will also make the eyes appear to be open wider. Flynn and coworkers reported this change to be well accepted by their patients, but lowering of the eyelid after blepharoplasty surgery is generally considered a complication to be avoided. Further, some patients who complain of 'bunching' of their lower eyelid with smiling or animation actually have either excess eyelid skin or a normal amount of eyelid skin that is compressed into a small area by the upward movement of the cheek associated with strong contraction of the zygomaticus muscles. These patients will not benefit significantly from BTX injection into the lower eyelid. Thus, a careful examination and discussion about realistic goals is needed prior to treatment.

Preparation of BTX solution

There has been much discussion about ideal preparation methods for BTX type A (BTX-A). Botulinun toxin is a lyophilized preparation that must be diluted with saline solution in preparation for injection. Most injectors choose to add 1–5 mL of normal saline per 100 units of toxin, although up to 10 mL of saline has been reported. Although preservative-free saline is the agent approved by the Food and Drug Administration, studies have demonstrated that preserved saline causes less discomfort without decreasing efficacy. Many injectors have thus switched to preserved saline when reconstituting BTX-A. While there are clearly no absolute rules when preparing BTX-A for periorbital injection, it is

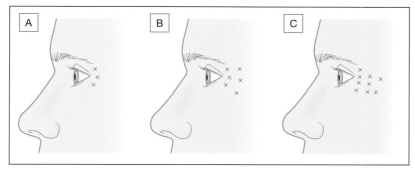

Fig. 5.8 (**A**) Typical lateral canthal injection pattern for treatment of dynamic rhytids in a patient with a small- to normal-sized orbicularis oculi muscle; 3–4 units of BTX-A are injected at each site. (**B**) Typical lateral canthal injection pattern for treatment of dynamic rhytids in a patient with a larger than normal orbicularis oculi muscle; 3–4 units of BTX-A are injected at each site. (**C**) Lateral canthal injection pattern that may be required in patients with a very large orbicularis oculi muscle. This type of injection scheme should only be administered by experienced injectors and is usually employed when a more conservative scheme has failed

easier for the novice injector to deliver very small doses (e.g. 1-unit increments) when working with a more dilute preparation. This may be helpful when only small amounts of toxin are to be injected in a given area. When larger amounts are needed, a more highly concentrated solution may be beneficial as the total volume injected can be minimized, thereby reducing the risk of diffusion into the orbit. The same concentration BTX-A solution may be used throughout the face and neck; it is not necessary to prepare a special dilution to treat the periorbital region. The dilutions used by the authors are 5 mL of sterile preserved saline per 100 Ut BTX-A (2 units in each 0.1 mL, KAA) and 2.5 mL of sterile preserved saline per l00 units BTX-A (4 units/0.1 mL, BB). Both authors deliver the injections from a 1-mL syringe with 30–32 gauge needle. The needles often need to be changed several times during a series of injections as the tips become dull quickly making the injections more difficult to administer, more painful for the patients, and more likely to induce ecchymosis as greater force is used to penetrate the tissue.

Dosage

Several authors have attempted to quantify the ideal dose of toxin. Blitzer et al used 2.5 units/injection site for a total of 5–15 units/side, depending on the distribution of facial lines. They used an EMG-injection technique to identify the muscle. Flynn recommends a dose of 12–15 units/side divided into three sites. Guerrissi described intraoperative injection of the orbicularis oculi muscle to treat crow's feet lines. In his first series he used between 15 and 50 units/muscle. In a follow-up series he injected 15 patients with a single intraoperative dose of 100 units per muscle.

The dosage of BTX-A injected into the periorbital region should be determined by the treatment goal, the size and strength of the orbicularis oculi muscle, and the position of the globe relative to the orbit. As detailed earlier, the size and distribution of the orbicularis oculi muscle may vary dramatically from patient to patient, and even within individuals from one side of the face to the other. Individuals with muscle distributed over a large area or with relatively hypertrophic muscle will require larger doses of toxin than may be considered 'standard.' Similarly, patients with smaller muscles that do not contract as forcefully should receive relatively lower doses of toxin. The dosage should also be reduced when injecting the lower eyelid and inferior lateral canthal region of patients with prominent globes due to shallow orbits, thyroid eye disease or myopia (extreme near-sightedness due to a longer than normal eye) as these patients are at higher risk for ectropion or incomplete eyelid closure. It is more helpful to think in terms of number of units per injection site than the total dose required to treat the entire region. As a general rule, 2.5–5 units/site is appropriate in the lateral canthal area. This will usually be injected into at least three, but up to ten, sites on each side of the face (see Fig. 5.8). When treating the inferior pretarsal orbicularis oculi muscle, only 1–2 units should be used per site (one or two sites per lower eyelid; see Fig. 5.10).

Injection technique

It is impossible to construct an injection site map or scheme that can be applied to patients in a generic manner. While some general guidelines can be applied, it is not feasible or appropriate to recommend a fixed number of injection sites, total dose of toxin, or the exact location of injection sites; treatments must be individualized to each patient. Asymmetry in orbicularis oculi muscle distribution often necessitates varying the dose of toxin between the two sides of the face. Figure 5.8 demonstrates some typical injection sites on patients with normal- and large-sized orbicularis oculi muscles. When injecting in the lateral canthal region, the risk of toxin diffusion into the orbit increases with proximity to the canthal angle. While there has yet to be a study to address this issue directly, it seems that injecting 1–1.5 cm from the lateral canthal angle minimizes the risk of clinical effects of toxin on the extraocular muscles.

Pain management techniques for periorbital BTX injections range from no anesthesia to the use of ice packs immediately prior to injection to the use of topical anesthetic agents. Extremely anxious patients may wish to take a benzodiazepine prior to injection but in this scenario transportation arrangements must be made as driving while sedated cannot be permitted. If a topical anesthetic agent is applied, it should be thoroughly removed prior to injection as the small 30 gauge needles will otherwise become occluded.

Brow contouring is covered extensively in Chapter 4. As the injections given to contour the brows are administered in the periorbital region, a few general comments in this chapter are warranted. First, injections given along the superior orbital rim should be performed with care. That is not to say injections cannot be safely given in this region. One of us (BSB) routinely treats patients with intractable blepharospasm injecting 5 units of BTX-A in each of three positions along the superior orbital rim (a total of 15 units) along with an additional 2.5–5 units in the medial and lateral portions of the upper eyelid itself (a total of 5–10 units), without adverse sequelae (Fig. 5.9). When injecting in this area, it is important to always direct the needle away from the

orbit as directing the toxin toward the eye may result in diffusion of toxin into extraocular muscles or even serious injury if the patient were to move suddenly during the injection. While difficult to study or prove definitively, the risk of toxin diffusion into the orbit may be reduced if the thumb of the nondominant (or noninjecting) hand is placed firmly along the orbital rim. The novice injector may wish to either stabilize their injecting hand against the patient, or their opposite, nondominant hand as it rests on the patient. This will prevent inadvertent perforation of veins or the eye in the event of an unexpected movement. When administering injections in the periorbital region, the injector must take great care to always point the needle away from the eye itself. To minimize the risk of ecchymosis, injections in this region are best administered intradermally or subcutaneously. When possible, injecting immediately over vessels should be avoided.

Although it is generally true that absolute rules about dosage and number of injection sites should not be made, great care should be taken when injecting the pretarsal orbicularis oculi muscle. This muscle can be injected in its central portion (immediately below the pupil) or alternately, may be injected in two sites, roughly corresponding to the medial and lateral corneoscleral limbus. If a single central injection is planned, a dose of no more than 2 units should be injected initially (Fig. 5.10). Additional injections can be administered as needed at the 2-week follow-up visit. If two separate sites are used, no more than 1–1.5 units should be delivered at each site. Excessive delivery of toxin in this region can impair eyelid closure and may lead to tearing, ectropion, and even inward turning of the eyelid against the eye (entropion). Entropion can

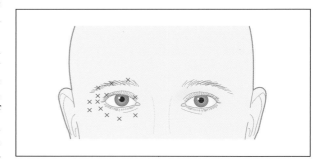

Fig. 5.9 Typical injection sites when treating benign essential blepharospasm; 2–5 units of toxin are injected at each site, including those in the upper eyelid. Total dose of BTX-A administered typically ranges from 25 to 75 units/side

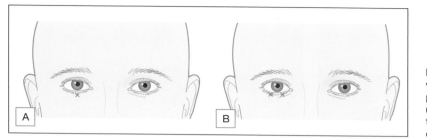

Fig. 5.10 (A) Typical injection sites when treating mild hypertrophy of the pretarsal orbicularis oculi muscle. **(B)** Typical injection sites when treating an even larger pretarsal orbicularis oculi muscle

occur when the preseptal orbicularis oculi muscle contracts forcefully in the setting of an immobile pretarsal muscle. In this situation the preseptal muscle moves upward overriding the pretarsal muscle and pushing the pretarsal muscle and eyelid margin inward toward the eye. This usually produces severe ocular pain and irritation. When administering lower eyelid injections, it is advisable to deliver the toxin subcutaneously to avoid diffusion into the inferior oblique muscle which occupies a relatively anterior position in the orbit. Injections should be administered from the side and never from in front of the patient to avoid having the needle directed towards the orbit. If the inferior oblique muscle is affected, vertical and/or torsional diplopia can result.

Complications of periocular BTX injection

As is generally the case, complications of BTX-A injections in the periorbital region may be related to the injection itself or to the toxin's effect. Complications of injection are usually related to pain and bruising. Although usually unnecessary, measures can be taken to minimize discomfort via the pretreatment use of ice, topical anesthetic preparations, or forced cold air (Zimmer Cryo 5, Zimmer Elektromedizin, Irvine, CA, USA). Prominent veins are often present in the lateral canthal region where they are prone to injury during injection. In an effort to avoid substantial ecchymosis and even hematoma formation, lateral canthal injections should be administered subcutaneously or even intradermally; intramuscular injections should be avoided. The clinical effects do not seem to be diminished by the more superficial injection site and the risk of hemorrhagic complications is reduced. Injection into the periorbital region (even into the upper eyelid itself) rarely causes eyelid ptosis. If ptosis does develop, it may be related to diffusion

of toxin into the levator muscle or, perhaps more commonly, to weakening of the frontalis muscle from concomitant forehead injection. In this latter situation, BTX injection uncovers a latent eyebrow ptosis which can no longer be adequately compensated by frontalis muscle action. In contrast, true eyelid ptosis caused by BTX effect on the levator muscle is characterized by normal eyebrow position, no change in the amount of dermatochalasis, and a low position of the eyelid relative to the superior corneoscleral limbus. It is important to distinguish between these mechanisms of ptosis as a ptotic eyelid often responds favorably to instillation of alpha-adrenergic eye drops (such as apraclonidine HCl), thus returning the lid to a normal position until the BTX effect is no longer evident. Alpha-adrenergic drops act via stimulation of Müller's muscle. It is possible to predict whether a patient will respond to apraclonidine drops by a simple test performed in the office. Several drops of apraclonidine HCl 0.5% or 1.0% (Iopidine, Alcon, Fort Worth, TX, USA), or phenylephrine hydrochloride 2.5% ophthalmic solution (Bausch and Lomb, Tampa, FL, USA) are placed in the affected eye. To ensure the best effect, the drops should be instilled beneath the upper eyelid as the patient gazes downward. This maneuver brings the drug in direct contact with the conjunctiva overlying Müller's muscle. Stimulation of this smooth muscle can elevate the upper eyelid by as much as 3 mm. The lower eyelid analog of Müller's muscle, the inferior tarsal muscle, is relatively poorly defined. Consequently, topical application of adrenergic agents does not produce significant change in lower eyelid position. In the event that eyelid ptosis develops after BTX injection, apraclonidine 0.5% drops may be used as necessary until the lid returns to an acceptable position, usually 2–4 weeks (Fig. 5.11).

Entropion and ectropion are rare complications of periorbital BTX injections. If they develop, an

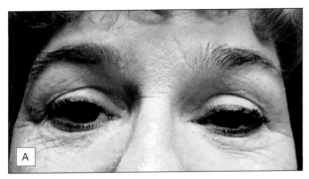
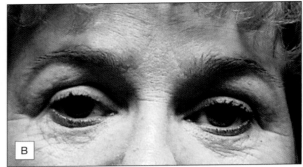

Fig. 5.11 (**A**) Left upper eyelid ptosis. (**B**) Ten minutes after instillation of apraclonidine HCl 0.5% in the left eye

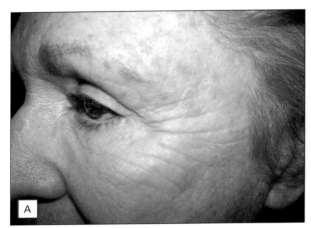
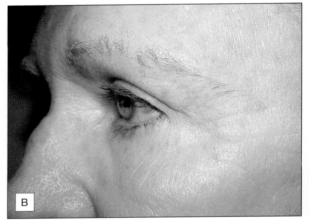

Fig. 5.12 (**A**) Patient with extensive photoaging and dynamic periorbital rhytids.(**B**) Same patient after full face intense pulsed light treatment and periorbital BTX-A injections (15 units)

ophthalmologist should be consulted for management to ensure that the ocular surface does not break down. As expected, these conditions are self-limited, usually resolving within 2–4 weeks. Tearing, lagophthalmos (incomplete eyelid closure), dry eye from diffusion of BTX into the lacrimal gland, and injury to the eye are all rare complications of periorbital BTX injection.

BTX and Adjunctive Treatments in Periorbital Rejuvenation

As alluded to earlier, stigmata of aging in the periorbital region include thinning of the skin, loss of elasticity, dyspigmentation, development of dermatochalasis on the eyelids, and descent of the eyebrows and midfacial structures. A comprehensive approach to periorbital rejuvenation typically includes not only BTX but also soft tissue fillers, chemical peels, ablative or nonablative laser skin resurfacing, intense pulsed treatment, and surgical modification of the forehead and eyebrows, eyelids, and/or midface. While clearly complementary to many other treatments, recent evidence suggests that BTX may actually act in a synergistic manner as well. Carruthers and Carruthers recently reported such an effect when BTX was used in combination with broadband light. The explanation for this synergism is not immediately clear but Carruthers and Carruthers postulate that it may be explained by BTX-A effects on autonomic vasodilation (Fig. 5.12). If BTX-A treatments are to be given to a patient undergoing eyelid surgery, it may be advisable to avoid injections in the lower eyelid or lateral canthus 1 week before and 2 weeks afterwards (Fig. 5.13). There have been anecdotal reports of facial muscle

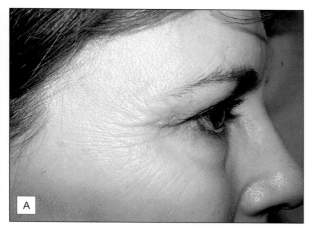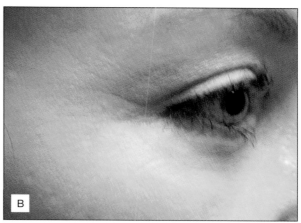

Fig. 5.13 (**A**) A 48-year-old female prior to BTX-A injection, CO_2 laser skin resurfacing, and upper and lower blepharoplasty. (**B**) Same patient, 12 weeks postoperatively

paralysis at a site distant from the BTX injection when surgery is performed less than 1 week after administration. As orbicularis oculi muscle contraction is felt to play an important role in forcing interstitial fluid into lymphatic drainage channels, it stands to reason that impairment of orbicularis muscle function may prolong the duration of postoperative swelling. BTX injections may be administered during the same treatment session as nonablative laser skin resurfacing, broadband light treatment, radiofrequency treatment, injection of soft tissue fillers, and other nonsurgical treatments.

Further Reading

Aguilar GL, Nelson C 1988 Eyelid and anterior orbital anatomy. In: Hornblass AH (ed) Oculoplastic, orbital and reconstructive surgery. Williams and Wilkins, Baltimore, pp. 4–22

American Society of Aesthetic Plastic Surgery Website [http://surgery.org/index.php]

Beard C 1985 Müller's superior tarsal muscle: anatomy, physiology, and clinical significance. Annals of Plastic Surgery 14:1324–1333

Bhawan J, Andersen W, Lee J, Labadie R, Solares G 1995 Photoaging versus intrinsic aging: a morphologic assessment of facial skin. Journal of Cutaneous Pathology 22(2):154–159

Biesman BS 1999 Anatomy of the eyelid, forehead, and temporal region. In: Biesman BS (ed) Lasers in facial aesthetic and reconstructive surgery. Williams and Wilkins, Baltimore, pp.15–27

Blitzer A, Binder WJ, Brin MF 2000 Botulinum toxin injections for facial lines and wrinkles: technique. In: Blitzer A, Binder WF, Boyd JB, Carruthers A (eds) Management of facial lines and wrinkles. Lippincott Williams and Wilkins, Philadelphia, pp. 303–313

Carruthers J, Carruthers A 2004 The effect of full-face broadband light treatments alone and in combination with bilateral crow's feet botulinum toxin type A chemodenervation. Dermatologic Surgery 30:355–366

Daniell HW 1971 Smoker's wrinkles: a study in the epidemiology of crow's feet. Annals of Intenal Medicine 75(6):873–880

Fagien S 1999 Botox for the treatment of dynamic and hyperkinetic facial lines and furrows: adjunctive use in facial aesthetic surgery. Plastic and Reconstructuve Surgery 103:701–708

Flynn TC 2003 Periocular botulinum toxin. Clinics in Dermatology 21:498–504

Flynn TC, Carruthers JA, Carruthers JA 2001 Botulinum-A toxin treatment of the lower eyelid improves infraorbital rhytids and widens the eye. Dermatologic Surgery 27(8):703–708

Goodman G 1998 Botulinum toxin for the correction of hyperkinetic facial lines. Australasian Journal of Dermatology 39(3):158–163

Guerrissi JO 2003 Intraoperative injection of botulinum toxin A into the orbicularis oculi muscle for the treatment of crow's feet. Plastic and Reconstructive Surgery 112(5 Suppl):161S–163S

Guerrissi JO, Sarkissian P 1997 Local injection into mimetic muscles of botulinum toxin A for the treatment of facial lines. Annals of Plastic Surgery 39:447–453

Kane MAC 2003 Classification of crow's feet patterns among Caucasian women: the key to individualizing treatment. Plastic and Reconstructive Surgery 112(5 Suppl):33S–39S

Schwartz RJ, Burns AJ, Rohrich RJ, Barton FE Jr, Byrd JS 1999 Long-term assessment of CO_2 facial laser resurfacing: aesthetic results and complications. Plastic and Reconstructive Surgery 103(2): 592–601

Singer M 1996 Botulinum toxin treatment of essential blepharospasm and hemifacial spasm. Ophthalmology 103(3):348

6 Botulinum Toxin in the Lips, Mid, and Lower Face

Roberta D. Sengelmann, Stacey Tull, Timothy C. Flynn

Introduction

The use of botulinum toxin type A (BTX-A) has been widely successful for the treatment of dynamic rhytides of the upper face. Based on the remarkable improvement in these wrinkles, BTX-A treatment has been expanded to other areas of the face. Although currently Food and Drug Administration (FDA)-approved only for the treatment of glabellar frown lines, physicians have developed numerous off-label indications which echo the success of this gold-standard treatment. Our understanding of the treatment of newer areas continues to expand.

BTX-A treatment of the lower face is now well understood. Whereas rhytides of the upper face are primarily dynamic, the lower face is subject to both dynamic as well as static forces. Dermatoheliosis, age-associated volume loss, and decreased resilience all contribute to the static rhytides. Not only does BTX-A aid in treating radial perioral rhytides (a.k.a. lipstick lines or sunbeam/smoker's wrinkles), but it also can soften the nasolabial and melolabial folds, lengthen the upper lip, or relax the chin. BTX-A is used both as a primary treatment modality and as an adjunct to other procedures aimed at rejuvenating the lower face.

BTX-A monotherapy is targeted to benefit patients with mild to moderate rhytides (Glogau II–III) whilst those with more severe rhytides often require combination therapy to elicit substantial clinical benefit. Common adjunctive procedures include dermal fillers, chemical peels, and laser resurfacing. This chapter will focus on BTX-A monotherapy and the chemodenervation aspect pertaining to these regimens; however, its use as an adjunct to volume replacement will also be mentioned (see Box 6.1).

Patient selection

As with all cosmetic procedures, patient selection is probably the most important factor contributing to a successful outcome. Patients must have reasonable expectations of what a particular procedure can or cannot achieve for them. Their expectations are developed in part through a successful preoperative evaluation and education experience with the physician. Many patients have had positive prior experiences with BTX-A (usually with treatment of the glabella and upper face) and are often interested in potential benefits for the lower face. The goal in treatment of the mid and lower face is to soften the wrinkles through muscular relaxation rather than to completely 'freeze' the target muscles and thus patients must realize that therapy is approached conservatively. This is especially true with initial treatments. Patients looking for dramatic changes may not be completely satisfied with BTX therapy

Areas of the mid and lower face amenable to BTX-A treatment	
Area	**Initial number of Botox units**
Radial lip rhytids	1–2 units each in four injections upper lip
Lip lengthening (gummy smile)	1 unit into each nasal facial groove
Nasolabial folds	1 unit into each nasal facial groove
Labiomental creases (marionette lines)	2–6 units each into depressor anguli oris
Chin softening (peach pit chin)	2–5 units into the mentalis muscle

Box 6.1 Areas of the mid and lower face amenable to BTX-A treatment

alone. Many patients are pleased with the use of BTX-A in combination with volume replacement. The highly functional nature of these areas (due to speaking and eating) may predispose the effects of BTX-A to wear off sooner than other areas. Some patients find this decreased length of effect prohibitive.

Patients also must consider how a particular result may affect their functionality and whether this would be an acceptable outcome. For instance, people who require precise enunciation such as public speakers or musicians who need tight control of their lips may find that treatment with perioral BTX-A leaves them with diminished ability to perform. Physicians must educate the patient about the effect of the musculature being treated and the conservative approach.

Treatment of the Mid and Lower Face

The complex and highly functional nature of the mid and lower face make this a more challenging area to treat. Not only do the muscles serve important functions such as oration, expression, and mastication, they are also synergistically interposed and closely intercalated with the superficial musculoaponeurotic system. For this reason, it is of utmost importance that the physician have a strong grasp of the regional anatomy and be well versed in the administration of BTX-A. Figure 6.1 illustrates the mid and lower facial musculature amenable to treatment. As this region is more prone to lend itself toward complications, it is strongly suggested that the novice hand become more comfortable with the more classically treated areas (i.e. the upper face) before attempting to tackle the lower face.

General technique

As with all cosmetic procedures, it is always good practice to obtain 'before' pictures with the patient in both static and dynamic poses. This is now easily accomplished with modern digital photography equipment. Having a separate area of the clinic which is used for pictures can ensure consistent lighting, and modern florescent bulbs can be obtained for use in this area which have a near daylight color balance. A fixed focal length lens also can serve to help with reproducible pictures by keeping the magnification and distance to the subject consistent. Storage of the digital files can be

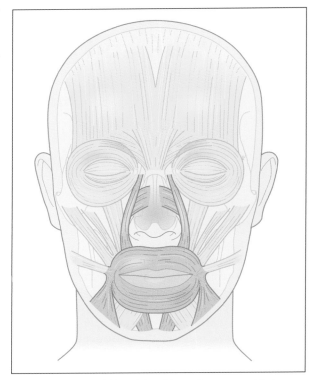

Fig. 6.1 Muscles of the mid and lower face amenable to treatment with botulinum toxin for cosmetic improvement

accomplished easily and cheaply using a computer for image storage or a central server that can store large amounts of image files inexpensively. Alternatively, pictures taken can be simply printed and placed in the patient's chart for reference at a later time. There is no substitute for good before and after clinical images in a cosmetic practice. With treatment of the mid and lower face, improvements may be subtle and reference to the pre- and post-treatment photographs may be needed to show the patient the degree of clinical improvement.

Informed consent should be signed, with the patient given ample opportunity to ask any questions they might have. Additionally, patients are encouraged to avoid the use of blood thinners for up to 2 weeks preoperatively, with permission from their primary care physician. These include prescribed medications such as warfarin (coumadin), anti-platelet medications (e.g. Plavix), and anti-inflammarory medications (e.g. Naprosyn, Voltaren), as well as over-the-counter medications and vitamin supplements. Patients can be asked specifically about the use of aspirin, nonacetominophen-based pain relievers (e.g. Advil, Aleve), vitamin E, St John's Wort, Ginkgo Biloba, and other herbs. Injections into highly vascular areas such as the lips can be associated with increased bruising in the patient using blood-thinning medications.

Prior to treatment, we suggest helping to visualize the target muscles by having the patient repeatedly contract and relax the area. After cleaning the area with an alcohol pad, we often mark the points of injection using a red nonpermanent 'dry erase' or water-soluble marker. We like to have the amount of BTX-A we plan to use drawn into the syringes, labeled, and placed on a procedure tray along with additional empty syringes, additional BTX-A, gauze, gloves, cotton tipped applicators, and ice packs.

Immediately prior to and following treatment to a given area, we have found it useful to have the patient place an ice pack on the target region. This has several benefits:

- it causes local vasoconstriction, which helps to prevent ecchymoses
- it has an anesthetic effect
- it creates a distraction for the patient.

We treat all patients in an electric exam table, seated in an upright position, and are prepared to recline them in case of a vasovagal response.

As always, precise injection technique into the chosen muscle is critical. The highly functional nature and higher risk for functional deficit associated with treating the lower face emphasizes this point. Diffusion away from the target site may be magnified if larger volumes and dilute concentrations of BTX-A are used.

Perioral rhytides

Radial perioral rhytides are caused in part by a hypertrophic orbicularis oris muscle, but are also exacerbated by age, sun exposure, and smoking. The orbicularis oris muscle functions as a sphincter which allows closure as well as protrusion of the lips, aiding mastication, expression, and phonation. These 'lipstick lines' or 'sunbeam/smoker's wrinkles,' as they are more commonly referred to, are found to be very unsightly for patients and pose a treatment challenge for clinicians.

Common methods to alleviate perioral rhytides include chemical peeling, laser resurfacing, and injection of filling agents. BTX-A serves to function either as monotherapy for mild–moderate rhytides

or is commonly used in conjunction with other procedures such as filler substances. The use of BTX-A in the perioral area prior to peeling or resurfacing can reduce the expression of these lines. This pretreatment can allow the patient to heal more smoothly and attain greater longevity of results. Concomitant use of a filler substance with BTX-A can improve the overall clinical effect by treating two components of the wrinkle: volume loss and hyperfunctional lines. This concomitant use has been shown to be synergistic in the glabella, and our experience substantiates this.

BTX-A as a monotherapy for the lips can be useful for those patients with minimal lines or for those patients desiring lip fullness. We have observed increased lip volume and slight upper lip eversion with BTX-A in the upper lip. This 'pseudoaugmentation' noted in many of our patients stems from the partial paresis of the orbicularis oris as a result of superficial placement of the injections. Figure 6.2 illustrates the increase in lip eversion with BTX monotherapy in the upper lip.

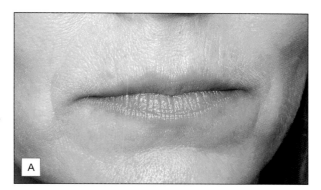

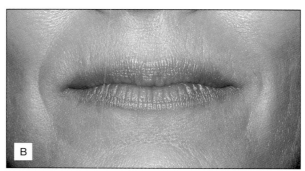

Fig. 6.2 (A) Before and **(B)** 2 weeks after 4 units (four injections of 1 unit each) of Botox is used in the upper lip. Note the increase in the amount of shown vermilion as well as lip eversion when 4 units are injected. With permission of Dermatologic Surgery

Treatment algorithm

As with all BTX-A treatments, dosage and placement of the injections are variable for each patient. We start by conservatively treating the upper lip, injecting 1–2 units at four evenly spaced sites along the vermilion border (refer to the diagram in Fig. 6.3). If the patient also has pronounced lower lip perioral rhytides, we inject 1–2 units at two evenly spaced sites along the lower vermilion border, approximately 1 cm medial to each oral commisure. We have the patients return for a follow-up visit in 2 weeks. If the initial procedure was well tolerated and the rhytides are still prominent, supplemental injections could be given. We also plan to treat more aggressively at the next session by adding two additional 1–2 units injections at the outer orbicularis of the upper lip and also possibly increasing the doses of injections at the vermilion border, depending on response.

We have found that results typically do not last as long as with treatment of the forehead and glabella. This may be in part due to the conservative doses used as limited data (see the article by Lowe) suggest that a dose-dependent relationship exists to some extent. An influential factor in treatment longevity may well be the continual use of the orbicularis oris in mouth functionality. In our practice, treatments are scheduled every 2–3 months to maintain optimal results.

Troubleshooting

As the goal of treatment in this area is rhytid reduction through subtle muscular paresis, it is paramount

that the patient be treated conservatively. This is in sharp contrast to injection techniques where a more complete muscular relaxation is the goal, such as with the glabellar complex. Start with minimal doses and base subsequent treatments on responsiveness. This can be most easily assessed by seeing the patient at a 2- to 3-week follow-up visit after initial treatment to gauge outcome and adjust dosage as necessary. In order to assure symmetry, care should be taken to mark the patient meticulously prior to injection and have a dosage plan made ahead of time. Additionally, in order to smooth rhytides whilst maintaining optimal functionality, injection depth should be limited to the most superficial layer of the orbicularis oris, just under the dermis.

Adverse effects and complications

After BTX-A treatment of perioral rhytides, especially with the upper lip, some patients have described difficulty associated with swishing and spitting, puckering, sipping from a straw, whistling or playing a brass or wind instrument, kissing, and with pronunciation of the letters 'p' and 'b'. One patient reported difficulty in using her mouth to eat soup with a spoon. We have found this sphincteric dysfunction to be dose-dependent and can be circumvented by adjusting the dosage, even by as little as 1 unit, with subsequent treatments. Patients with thin, atrophic upper lips or those with a long columella-to-vermilion distance can display an unattractive accentuation of these attributes with perioral BTX-A injection when treatment is too robust. Such patients may be more suited to combination therapy with lip augmentation. Finally, asymmetry is a potential complication that can best be prevented with careful, conservative planning and can be corrected at a follow-up visit if necessary.

Combination treatment of the lip with filler substances

One of the most common uses of BTX-A in our practices is in combination with filler substances. Many patients concerned with radial lip lines are experiencing age-associated volume loss. In order to achieve their desired degree of improvement, they need volume replacement of the perioral area. This can be accomplished with a number of filler substances, but the most common soft tissue fillers used for lip augmentation are injectable collagen or

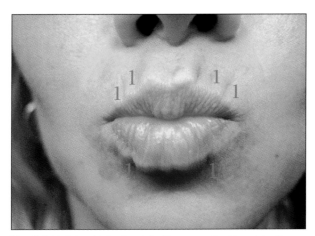

Fig. 6.3 Points of injection into the upper lip. Four injections of 1 unit of Botox is suggested as a starting point to decrease the appearance of radial lip lines

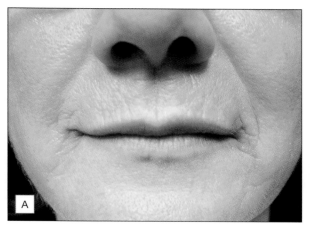 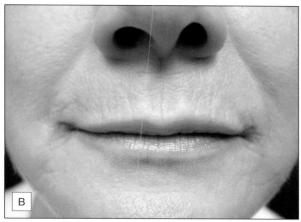

Fig. 6.4 Before and after pictures of a patient who had lip augmentation using both BTX-A and hyaluronans. Restylane was used as the filler

hyaluronans. Lip volume replacement can be achieved by vermilion border being accentuated or expansion of the pink portion of the lip. Beyond stretching these lines out through volume enhancement, the discrete radial lip lines themselves can also be targeted with superficial filler placement. BTX-A can assist in improving the appearance of the lips by relaxing the hypertrophic orbicularis muscle, which further softens rhytids and allows a pseudoaugmentation. The sequence of this combination therapy varies according to the preference of the physician and patient tolerance. For example, if collagen is to be injected into the lips, it makes sense to treat with BTX-A thereafter as the lidocaine in the filler will improve patient comfort. But in the case where nerve blocks are to be performed before hyaluronic acid treatment, then the sequence of events is less critical. Figure 6.4 shows improvement when filler substances and BTX-A are used as a combination approach.

Lip lengthening
Patients

When the upper lip retracts abnormally high due to contraction of the levator labii superioris alaquae nasi (LLSAN) (see Fig. 6.5), patients are left with a 'gummy smile.' This results in the unflattering exposure of the bases of the canines and upper incisors as well as the entire upper gumline. Injection of BTX-A into the LLSAN at this site will cause partial paresis and allow lengthening of the upper lip so that the smile does not expose as much of the

gingiva. Figure 6.6 shows improvement with the use of BTX-A for lip lengthening.

Treatment algorithm

Once again, in such a highly functional zone, care must be taken to treat conservatively. Begin conservatively by injecting 1 unit at the nasofacial groove into each levator complex, as shown in Figure 6.7. The muscle and injection site target can be determined by placing a fingertip on the pyriform aperture just inferior to the nasomaxillary groove. As opposed to the multiple superficial injections of BTX-A into the orbicularis oris, injection of the LLSAN is placed as a single dose just above periosteum. A 2- to 3-week follow-up is recommended, with subsequent dose modification guided by clinical response. Dr Michael Kane, a plastic surgeon with over 14 years of experience treating this area, may inject up to 5 units at each site. Upper lip augmentation with fillers may also aid in camouflaging the upper gumline and bases of the teeth.

Troubleshooting

Care must be taken to perform this technique on appropriate candidates. Patients with 'Mona Lisa' smiles, where the oral commissures naturally fall below the upper lip, can be further exaggerated by BTX-A injections at this site and lead to an unnatural appearance. Alternatively, patients with upper and lower gummy show may require concomitant treatment of the depressor labii inferioris to avoid a

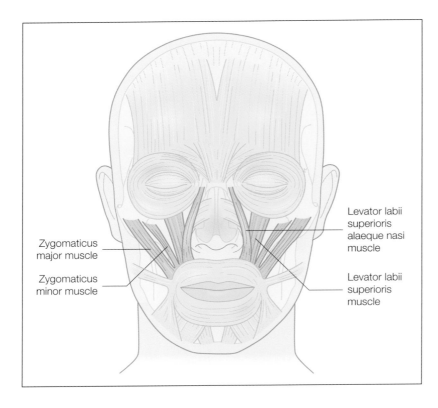

Zygomaticus
major muscle

Zygomaticus
minor muscle

Levator labii
superioris
alaeque nasi
muscle

Levator labii
superioris
muscle

Fig. 6.5 The LLSAN, levator labii superioris, and zygomaticus major and minor muscles are shown in this anatomic drawing

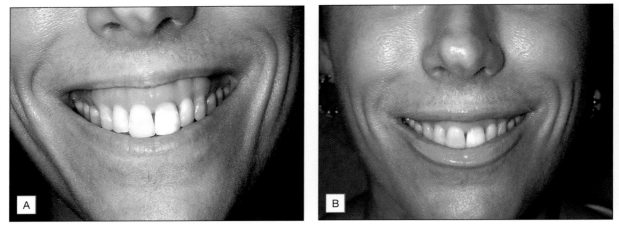

Fig. 6.6 Improvement in the degree of gummy smile achievable through treatment of the levator labii superioris alaeque nasi. Relaxation of the muscle reduces the degree of travel of the upper lip and results in a functional lengthening of the lip. (**A**) Pre-Botox for gummy smile. (**B**) 20 days after Botox for LLSAN to treat gummy smile

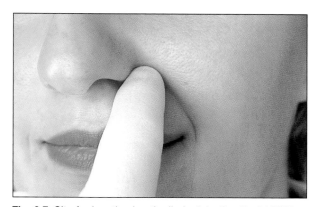

Fig. 6.7 Site for lengthening the lip by injecting the LLSAN. Injections are performed bilaterally. A finger on the piriform aperture can help identify the injection site

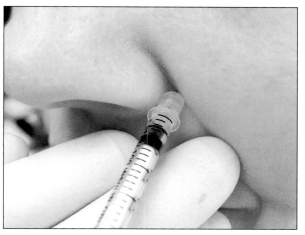

Fig. 6.8 Injection of the LLSAN muscle is done at the juncture of the nasofacial groove

grimacing smile that may be a consequence of treating only the LLSAN.

Adverse effects and complications

Potential risks associated with treatment of the LLSAN include overtreatment causing upper lip ptosis, excessive lengthening, lower lip protrusion, and the potential for asymmetrical results. Excessive lengthening can occur to the extent that the patient appears edentulous.

Nasolabial folds

Patients

For patients with mild to moderate nasolabial fold accentuation, BTX-A monotherapy can be of great benefit. Young to middle-aged patients typically in their 30s to 50s are ideal candidates because the etiology of their prominent nasolabial folds is muscular in nature. In contrast, older patients typically have more extensive dermatoheliosis and skin laxity, which allows for descent of malar fat pads and a distinct groove at the nasolabial fold. This is further accentuated by the natural lipoatrophy of the upper lip which comes with age. Such patients may be better served with more aggressive treatments for prominent nasolabial folds such as soft tissue fillers or implants and mid face lifts.

Treatment of prominent nasolabial folds with BTX-A remains a controversial subject. Some clinicians prefer to treat the levator labii superioris alaquae nasi (LLSAN), while others prefer to treat the zygomaticus muscles. In our experience, we have found that treatment of the LLSAN with BTX-A to be more effective in treating the most superior and medial portions of the nasolabial fold. While injection of the zygomaticus muscles can effectively flatten prominent nasolabial folds, care must be taken not to treat at the expense of causing a disfigured smile (Fig. 6.8).

Treatment algorithm

Treatment of the LLSAN for prominent nasolabial folds follows the protocol as outlined above for lip lengthening.

Troubleshooting

Only patients with smiles that are amenable to lip lengthening as an associated result should be treated with BTX-A injection to the LLSAN. Additionally, careful patient selection and reasonable patient expectations are both crucial considerations. As with treatment of perioral rhytides, treatment of more pronounced nasolabial folds with BTX-A may be best as adjunctive therapy rather than monotherapy. In this way, more dramatic results can be achieved without the greater risk for functional compromise associated with higher doses of BTX-A. As shown in the study by deMaio, temporary dermal filling agents seem to have a longer tissue residence time and clinical benefit when administered with BTX-A. This may be due to the more static nature of the tissue thereafter and slowed catabolism.

Adverse effects and complications

Upper lip ptosis has been reported as a potential side effect of BTX-A treatment for periorbital rhytides as a result of diffusion into the zygomaticus muscles. Not surprisingly, this poses a stronger threat when purposefully injecting into the zygomatic muscles to achieve flattening of the nasolabial folds. Conservative and cautious treatment of this area will help to prevent such a complication. Care must be taken to avoid injecting below the zygomatic arch and deeply into the zygomaticus major, which is primarily responsible for elevation of the upper lip and mouth. Such a mistake can cause drooping of the lateral aspect of the mouth, giving the impression of having a Bell's palsy. Unlike upper-eyelid ptosis caused by diffusion of BTX-A into the levator palpebrae superioris muscle which usually lasts about 3 weeks and can be palliated with eye drops that stimulate Müllers muscle, upper lip and mouth ptosis takes longer to resolve (about 6 weeks) and has no 'antidote' or treatment to speed recovery of function.

Labiomental creases

Patients

The downward 'drool grooves' at the angles of the mouth and their extension to the lateral mentum creating 'marionette lines' are caused by the action of the depressor anguli oris muscle. Such an appearance can be disconcerting to the patient as it creates a permanent look of anger and frustration. Severe cases can also predispose toward angular cheilitis. Partial paresis of this muscle can allow the zygomaticus muscles to elevate more effectively the corners of the mouth, resulting in a more pleasant, approving appearance. Additionally, treatment of the depressor anguli oris in conjunction with dermal fillers can greatly reduce the appearance of more prominent marionette lines (Fig. 6.9).

Treatment algorithm

The depressor anguli oris is shaped like a triangle with its vertex located at the angle of the mouth (Fig. 6.10). Optimal results with BTX-A are

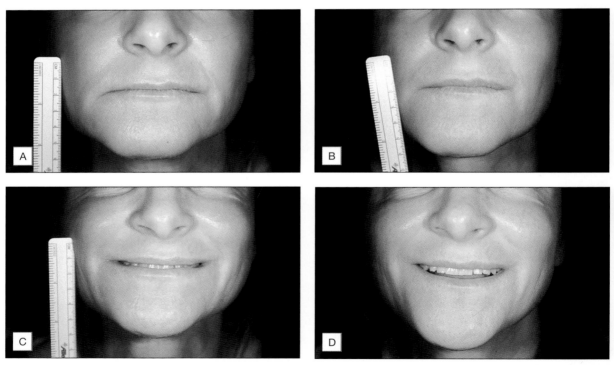

Fig. 6.9 Before and after improvements are shown with injection of the depressor anguli oris muscle. Note elevation of the corners of the mouth and the increased smile

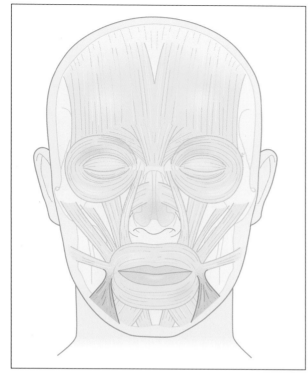

Fig. 6.10 The depressor anguli oris muscle is a triangular muscle with its base originating at the mandible

achieved by injecting into the mid and lower thirds of the muscle where it is closely intertwined with fibers of the platysma which also exert pull at the corners of the mouth. A conservative approach is recommended and might include injecting 1–2 units at each site bilaterally. We recommend re-evaluating at a 2- to 3-week follow-up, and adjusting the dose as indicated up to a total of 4–7.5 units/side. All injection points should be lateral to the oral commisure to prevent diffusion into depressor labii inferioris, which would result in lip protrusion.

Troubleshooting

Once again, patients should be carefully selected based on anticipation of reasonable results. The goal of monotherapy is to lift the corners of the mouth slightly. Many patients have such severely prominent lines in this area that BTX-A should be considered as an adjunct to soft tissue augmentation. Filler substances are commonly used in this area to expand the indented corners of the mouth. Hyaluronans and collagens work well to lift this

area. If the patient desires the maximum benefit to the mouth corners, a combination approach with fillers and BTX-A can be employed.

Adverse effects and complications

As we have discussed with all BTX-A injections of mid and lower face dynamic rhytides, the highly functional nature of these areas demands that we proceed with caution. Placement of an injection too medially may lead to diffusion into the depressor labii inferioris muscles, resulting in protrusion of the lower lip and an appearance akin to 'Gomer Pile.' Additionally, care must be taken to avoid inadvertently causing paresis of the buccinator muscle by injection too laterally which would predispose the patient to biting and traumatizing their buccal mucosa. Placement of injections at the inferiormost aspect of depressor anguliI oris along the mandible can help reduce the risk of adverse effects while still bringing on a subtle upturning of the corners of the mouth and an esthetically pleasing result.

Chin softening
Patients

Patients with hyperfunctional mentalis muscles create the appearance of an 'apple dumpling deformity' or a 'peach pit' chin. This occurs mostly with expression and may represent excessive innervation of the musculature or habit contraction. Some patients have a very active mentalis with talking and the excessive movement of the chin can be an unattractive distraction. The deformity can also be seen at rest, especially as advancing age predisposes us to loss of dermal collagen and subcutaneous fat, further exposing underlying musculature. Atrophic acne scarring in this area can accentuate this unsightly appearance. Depending on the extent and etiology of the defect, injection with BTX-A can be used either alone or in conjunction with soft tissue augmentation. Indeed, patients are frequently seen for perioral soft tissue augmentation not realizing that treatment of the mentalis and depressor anguli oris can give a softer and more relaxed appearance. Additionally, patients with clefting of the chin who do not like this appearance due to muscular diastasis may achieve a smoother result with BTX-A injections, especially in combination with filling agents (Fig. 6.11).

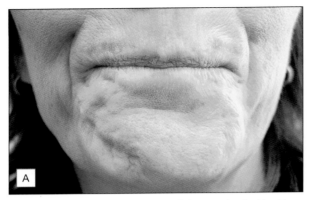
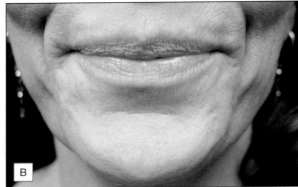

Fig. 6.11 Before and after photos of the peach pit chin. Five units of Botox were injected into the point of the chin to improve appearance

Treatment algorithm

For patients without clefting of the chin, we initially treat by injecting 2.5–5 units of BTX-A at the mental protuberance (Fig. 6.12). Patients with clefted chins require two injections of 2.5–5 units at each site in order to treat each muscle 'belly' effectively. A total of 10 units, and rarely as much as 15 units, can be used to treat the entire muscle complex given as one or two injections.

Troubleshooting

An interesting note is that many patients will not necessarily be aware of the peach pit chin or excessive movement of the mentalis while talking, but following successful treatment will often return and ask that the area be retreated. They often comment that they had not appreciated the significant improvement that is possible with mentalis treatment. The dose of BTX-A required is relatively low and easy to deliver, with a reproducible and excellent response. Injection into the central to lower portion of the mentalis reduces the risk of affecting the orbicularis oris muscle and causing undesired lip prolems.

Adverse effects and complications

When treating the mentalis, and especially when delivering larger doses (<10 units) and more laterally placed injections to treat clefting, care must be taken to avoid inadvertently causing paresis of the depressor labii inferioris as well as orbicularis oris which may affect speech or sphincteric function.

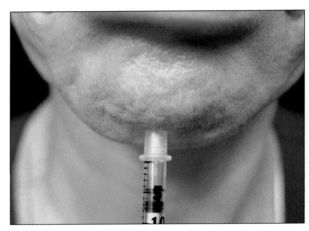

Fig. 6.12 Injection of the mentalis muscle can be accomplished in most patients with just a single injection into the central portion of the muscle

Conclusion

Treatment of the muscles of the mid and lower face which contribute to dynamic rhytides is among the newest arsenal in the off-label use of BTX-A. The physician must take great care to understand the functional anatomy of this region in order to clearly comprehend the benefits, limitations, and potential side effects of chemodenervation with BTX-A treatment. Only then can the physician accurately convey reasonable expectations to their patients. Because of the highly functional nature of these target muscles, a conservative and cautious treatment approach cannot be overemphasized. More often than not, BTX-A for the mid and lower face is used adjunctively with filling agents and other rejuvenation techniques and, rarely, is it used as monotherapy.

Further Reading

Alam M, Dover JS, Klein AW, Arndt KA 2002 Botulinum A exotoxin for hyperfunctional facial lines: where not to inject. Archives of Dermatology 138:1180–1185

Carruthers J, Carruthers A 2001 BOTOX use in the mid and lower face and neck. Seminars in Cutaneous Medicine and Surgery 20:85–92

de Maio M 2003 Botulinum toxin in association with other rejuvenation methods. Journal of Cosmetic and Laser Therapy 5(3–4):210–212

Defazio G, Abbruzzese G, Girlanda P, et al 2002 Botulinum toxin A treatment for primary hemifacial spasm: a 10-year multicenter study. Archives of Neurology 59(3):418–420

Kane MA 2003 The effect of botulinum toxin injections on the nasolabial fold. Plastic and Reconstructive Surgery 112(5 Suppl): 66s–72s

Lowe NJ, Lask G, Yamauchi P, Moore D 2002 Bilateral, double-blind, randomized comparison of 3 doses of botulinum toxin type A and placebo in patients with crow's feet. Journal of the American Academy of Dermatology 47(6):834–840

Matarasso SL, Matarasso A 2001 Treatment guidelines for botulinum toxin type A for the periocular region and a report on partial upper lip ptosis following injections to the lateral canthal rhytides. Plastic and Reconstructive Surgery 108:208–214

Papel ID, Capone RB 2001 Botulinum toxin A for mentalis muscle dysfunction. Archives of Facial Plastic Surgery 3:268–269

Semchyshyn N, Sengelmann RD 2003 Botulinum toxin A treatment of perioral rhytides. Dermatologic Surgery 29:490–495

Sposito MM 2002 New indications for botulinum toxin type A in cosmetics: mouth and neck. Plastic and Reconstructive Surgery 110:601–611

Sposito MM 2002 New indications for botulinum toxin type A in treating facial wrinkles of the mouth and neck. Aesthetic Plastic Surgery 26:89–98

7

Neck Treatment

Frederic Brandt, Andres Boker, Brent R. Moody

Introduction

The aging neck is increasingly recognized for its esthetic importance. Physicians can offer a number of surgical and nonsurgical options for neck rejuvenation. The critical step in neck rejuvenation is the proper evaluation of the pathologic process in each individual. A thorough understanding of the various components of neck aging allows the physician to select the appropriate therapy or combination of therapies.

Botulinum toxin (BTX) chemodenervation revolutionized cosmetic surgery. In many cases, invasive surgical procedures are supplanted or augmented through the use of BTX. At the conclusion of this chapter, the reader will understand the proper utilization of BTX in neck rejuvenation.

Neck aging

The pathophysiology of the aging neck involves multiple factors that culminate in an esthetically undesirable appearance. The skin itself is subject to degenerative changes: loss and disorder of collagen and elastin. External factors, primarily ultraviolet radiation exposure, lead to further aberrations in the skin's connective tissue matrix. Ultraviolet exposure also creates vascular changes leading to Poikiloderma of Civatte. Deleterious alterations in the extracellular matrix combined with the downward vector effect of gravity leads to sagging of both skin and the underlying platysmal muscle.

Changes in the platysma that have been described as hypertrophic lead to characteristic platysmal bands. This apparent hypertrophy of the muscle is likely a clinical finding rather than a true muscle hypertrophy. Hypertrophy of a muscle occurs from an increase in the cross-sectional myofiber diameter and resultant muscle mass. The mechanisms driving muscle hypertrophy are not fully understood, but remain under active investigation. Current literature lacks detailed histologic studies comparing platysmal bands versus nonbanded platysma. The clinical entity we call platysmal banding most likely results from separation of the normally decussated muscle. As these anterior bands of the platysma separate, they may assume a tightened appearance.

Fat accumulation and fat repositioning in the subcutaneous and subplatysmal planes leads to localized adiposity. With aging, new adipose tissue can accumulate in the submental region, just as it can in any other body location. A fat repositioning leading to a pseudo-excess of submental fat can also develop. As the platysma loses integrity and separates in the midline, the muscular buttress holding the subplatysmal fat fails and the fat descends, becoming clinically apparent. A useful categorization for degenerative changes in the neck has been developed (Fig. 7.1).

Overall, the aging neck can display one or more of these features: vascular and pigmentary alteration, platysmal bands, skin laxity, and adipose accumulation. Treatment options exist for each of these changes. Table 7.1 highlights treatment options for neck rejuvenation. To achieve optimal improvement, a combination of modalities may be required. Lasers and light-based therapies are successful in the treatment of Poikiloderma of Civatte. Liposuction can address subcutaneous excess adiposity. Open dissection can remove the subplatysmal fat pad. Sagging of the platysma can be managed surgically through techniques such as corset platysmoplasty. It is the platysmal bands and horizontal 'necklace' lines that are most amenable to BTX therapy.

Anatomy

The platysma is generally considered the inferior-most portion of the superficial musculoaponeurotic

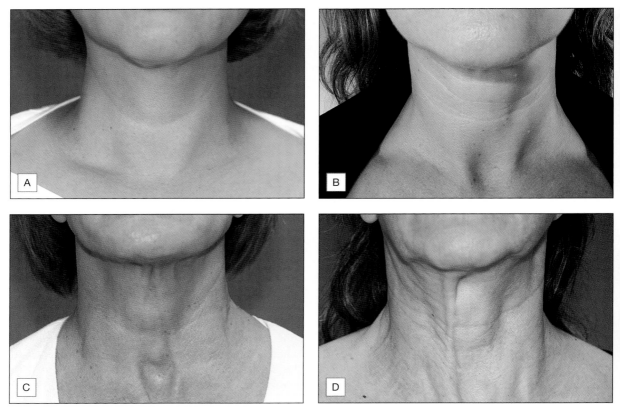

Fig. 7.1 Categories of age-related neck degeneration

Treatment options for neck rejuvenation		
Condition	**Nonsurgical management**	**Surgical management**
Poikiloderma of Civatte	Pulsed dye laser, Intense pulsed light	None
Adipose accumulation	BTX in type II platysmal anatomy	Liposuction, lipectomy
Platysmal bands	BTX	Platysmoplasty (various techniques)
Horizontal 'necklace lines'	BTX	+/− neck lift
Excess skin	Radiofrequency for lateral neck	Neck lift

Table 7.1 Treatment options for neck rejuvenation

system (SMAS). While some recent anatomic investigations question the extent of the SMAS, most evidence points to its existence as both an anatomic entity and a surgically relevant concept. The platysma is a broad sheet-like muscle surrounded by its own fascia layer overlying the cervical fascia. The muscle originates inferiorly as two independent sheets from the upper chest, with connections to the fascia overlying the pectoralis and deltoid muscles. The muscle courses anteriomedially with fibers even-tually blending with the following facial muscles: masseter, depressor anguli oris, mentalis, risorius, and the orbicularis oris. This intimate relationship of the platysma and the musculature of the lower face allows the platysma to contribute not only to neck aging but descent of the lower face as well. Some surgeons propose that the SMAS is better considered as the platysma aponeurosis and is confluent with the muscles of the midface, including the zygomaticus major and the orbicularis oculi. This

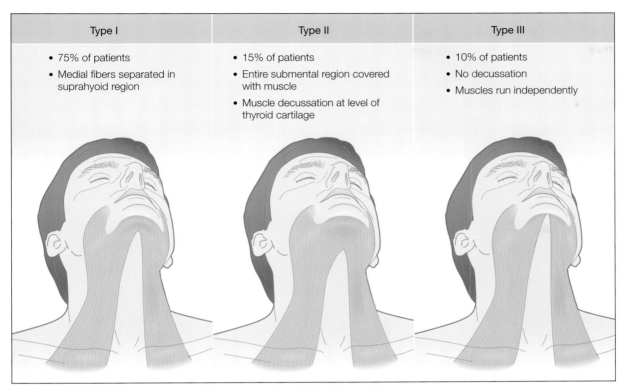

Type I	Type II	Type III
• 75% of patients • Medial fibers separated in suprahyoid region	• 15% of patients • Entire submental region covered with muscle • Muscle decussation at level of thyroid cartilage	• 10% of patients • No decussation • Muscles run independently

Fig. 7.2 Variants of platysma anatomy. (Adapted from Brandt FS, Boker A 2003 Botulinum toxin for rejuvenation of the neck. Clinics in Dermatology 21:513–520)

concept serves to further underscore the importance of neck management in any comprehensive rejuvenation attempt.

The medial fibers of the platysma exhibit considerable anatomic variation and are most responsible for the aged appearance of the neck. As illustrated in Figure 7.2, three anatomic variations have been described. The type I variant is seen in approximately three out of four individuals. In this variant, the platysmal fibers interdigitate with the contralateral muscular fibers at a level approximately 1–2 cm submentally. In the type II variant, seen in approximately 15% of patients, the fibers meet at the level of the thyroid cartilage. This provides a covering of the entire submental region. In 10% of cases, a third variant will be found. In this situation, the fibers do not interdgitate at all, but rather insert independently.

Esthetically important fat in the neck occurs subcutaneously as the submental fat pad and as subplatysmal fat. The superficial submental fat is amenable to removal via tumescent liposuction, whereas the subplatysmal fat is extractable only through open surgical approaches. However, nonsurgical improvement in fat pads is achievable through BTX injection. In patients with type II platysmal anatomy, relaxing the platysma bands with BTX will allow unopposed contraction of the fibers overlying the fat pad and therefore apply vertical pressure onto the fat pad.

Germane platysmal and subplatysmal anatomy is presented in Figure 7.3. As BTX injections in the platysma are superficial, the likelihood of inadvertent injection into a deeper structure is low. The motor innervation of the platysma comes from the cervical branch of the facial nerve. The sensory innervation of the neck arises from branches of the cervical plexus.

Rejuvenation of the Neck

Patients seeking esthetic improvement of the neck generally present with one or more of the problems described above: Poikiloderma of Civatte, skin laxity, horizontal 'necklace' lines, vertical platysma bands, or submental fullness. When assessing

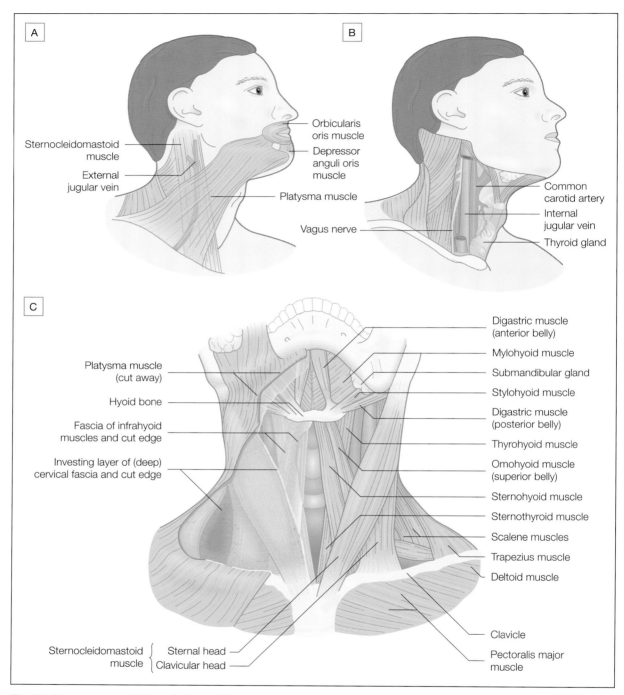

Fig. 7.3 Neck anatomy. (**A**) Superficial and (**B**) deep anatomical relations of the neck. (**C**) Anterior view of the muscles of the neck

patients for potential cosmetic treatments of the neck, we favor starting the consultation visit with a broad, open-ended question such as 'What about your neck would you like improved?' Many times patients will ask the physician what should be done, placing the physician in the awkward position of imposing their own esthetic value judgment onto the patient. By encouraging the patient to verbalize their expectations, patients demonstrate that they have contemplated their goals. It is often helpful for patients to bring photographs of themselves at a younger age. This exercise may help the physician in understanding the patient's goals. If the patient has realistic expectations and the physician feels that these expectations can be met with an acceptable safety profile, the likelihood of success is maximized.

Fortunately, BTX injections are extremely safe and absolute contraindications to its use are few. Neck injection may not be prudent in patients with a history of neck weakness or dysphagia. Additionally, patients with chronic neck pain should be treated with caution as muscular weakness may be an etiology in this condition. After assessing the patient's goals and reviewing the medical history, a focused physical examination with the patient in the upright position is performed. Key elements of the exam include an assessment of vertical platysmal bands, horizontal neck rhytids, skin laxity, submental fat, jowls, and overall mandibular contour. The examination should be performed with the patient at rest and with the anterior neck contracted. After performing the examination, the physician places the patient into the appropriate category of age-related neck degeneration.

Patient selection for BTX neck rejuvenation and treatment protocol

Patients with category II and III neck aging are most satisfied with BTX neck rejuvenation. Additionally, patients who are not suitable surgical candidates, and prior face or neck lift patients who do not desire further surgical intervention, are potential candidates for BTX neck rejuvenation. Experienced clinicians have noted that younger patients as well as prior facelift patients do particularly well.

Clinicians should use the BTX dilution with which they are most familiar. Our preferred dilution of BTX-A (Botox, Allergan Inc., Irvine, CA, USA) is 2.0 mL of preserved normal saline per 100-unit vial, yielding a concentration of 50 units of Botox/mL.

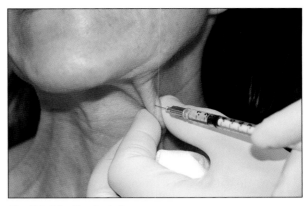

Fig. 7.4 Injection technique

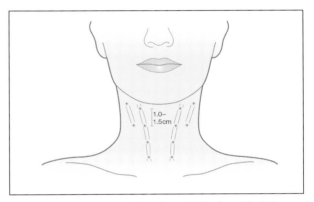

Fig. 7.5 Locations of typical points of injection of botulinum toxin into the platysma muscle

Injection occurs with a half-inch 30 gauge needle attached to a 1 cc syringe (1 cc syringes are commercially available with 50 gradation marks per syringe, allowing for precise dosing at 1 unit of Botox per gradation mark).

The patient is asked to contract their anterior neck by clenching their teeth and depressing the lateral oral commissures. This maneuver will exaggerate the platysmal bands. Using the nondominant hand, the physician stabilizes the band by holding the band between the thumb and index finger. The physician inserts the needle into the platysmal band. With experience, the injecting physician will learn to identify the resistance of the platysma muscle. Once this resistance is met, the correct injection depth is located. Figure 7.4 illustrates the injection technique. Injections of 3–10 units are placed into the platysmal band at 1.0- to 1.5-cm intervals from the jawline to the lower neck. Figure 7.5 demonstrates typical injection locations. Thinner bands will respond to 15–20 units of toxin, while thicker bands may require up to 30 units. A total dose of 50–100 units is delivered. While use of higher doses of Botox have been reported in the neck, concern for side effects such as platysmas and sternomastoid weakness and dysphagia increases.

Horizontal neck rhytids, commonly referred to as necklace lines, are also amenable to chemodenervation. Injection of 1–2 units at 1-cm intervals along the rhytid will reduce or eliminate the line. For these lines, the injection is intradermal. There is concern that deeper injection may weaken musculature necessary for swallowing.

Our experience with BTX-B (Myobloc, Allergan Inc., Irvine, CA) for rejuvenation of the neck has been limited to use in clinical trials. In our most recent study, 15 patients were randomized to three different treatment groups according to dose (2500 units, 5000 units, and 7500 units). The design was based on a 100 : 1 conversion rate for dose equivalence to Botox Cosmetic. The mean onset of action of platysma muscle paralysis and achievement of the desired cosmetic result was at 2.8 days. Patients in the 2500 units group did not report any adverse reactions; however, only two patients reported having a cosmetic improvement. Out of the 10 patients within the intermediate- to high-dose groups, eight reported moderate to severe dry mouth as the most bothersome side effect. All of them had a significant esthetic improvement and regressed at leased one point in the Platysmal Band Prominence Scale (primary end point of the study). The mean duration of effect was 13.2 weeks and was directly proportional to the total dose injected.

In summary, we can conclude that BTX-B has comparable clinical efficacy to BTX-A (Botox Cosmetic), maybe even showing an earlier onset of action. However, its increased adverse reactions profile and possibly shorter duration of effect is likely to restrict its use to patients who have previously been nonresponsive to the A serotype.

Other commercial sources of BTX-A such as Dysport (Inamed, Santa Barbara, CA, USA) have not been specifically tested for neck rejuvenation in a controlled clinical trial setting. However, anecdotal data from European practices points to close similarities to Botox Cosmetic in terms of onset of action and virtual absence of adverse reactions.

Anesthetic requirements are negligible. In many cases, none is required. For anxious or particularly sensitive patients, topical anesthetics or preinjection application of a cold pack can be utilized. The use of a 30-gauge needle will provide less discomfort than the use of larger bore needles.

BTX can improve the chest wall as well. Women may exhibit wrinkling of the so-called décolleté of the central mid chest. BTX has been successfully utilized to reduce these wrinkles (Fig. 7.6). The described technique involves injections occurring in a nearly vertical line just superior to the line of

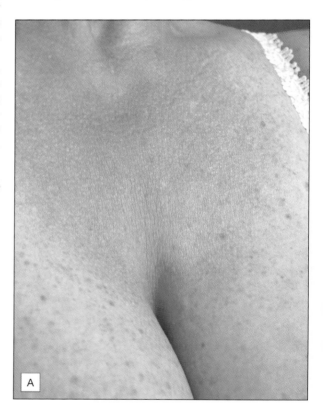

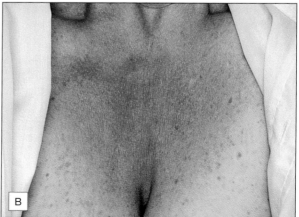

Fig. 7.6 Décolleté

maximal wrinkling upon contraction. Approximately six injections of 3–4 units per injection at 2-cm intervals are performed. Horizontal lines are treated by injecting in a V-shaped pattern with its point at the presternal region. A total of eight injections of 3–4 units per injection at 2-cm intervals are performed in the central chest. A single report has described BTX injections to mitigate anterior chest wall and neck flushing.

Results

Results of treatment are typically noted at 5–7 days postinjection. Results may take up to 14 days, therefore reinjection is not recommended before this time. In patients with category II or III neck degenerative changes, 98.5% had good to excellent results as judged by the patients and physicians. Patients with the most severe banding were less likely to report improvement. Significant skin excess may decrease the overall esthetic benefit. Pretreat-

ment degree of flaccidity and hypertrophy are the most important determinants of success. Figures 7.7–7.9 illustrate clinical examples.

Sequelae include reactions from the injections themselves. Edema, erythema, bruising, muscle soreness, and neck discomfort are the most common occurrences. No significant alteration in the patient's skin care regimen is required. Patients are asked not to massage or rub the injection area for 24 hours. Additionally, patients are cautioned against lying flat on their back for the first 4 hours after injection.

Complications are fortunately rare. Dysphagia has been observed. It is felt that dysphagia results from toxin spread to the underlying muscles of deglutination. While the dose to induce dysphagia has generally felt to be high (mean of 184 units), one patient has been reported to develop profound dysphagia requiring the use of a nasogastric feeding tube after the use of 60 units of Botox. Neck weakness can also result from treatment. This generally manifests as difficulty with neck flexion while in

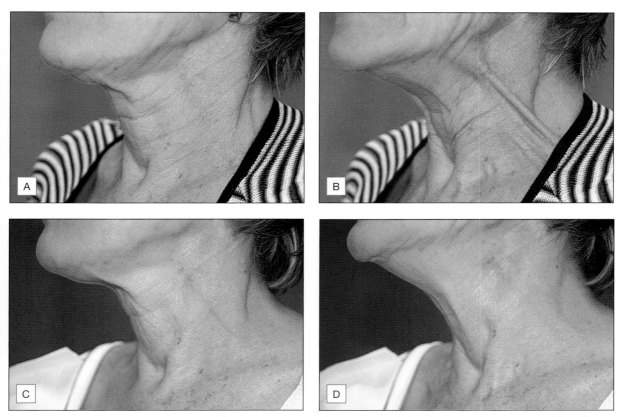

Fig. 7.7 (**A**) Neck at rest before treatment, (**B**) neck contracted before treatment, (**C**) neck at rest after treatment, (**D**) neck contracted after treatment

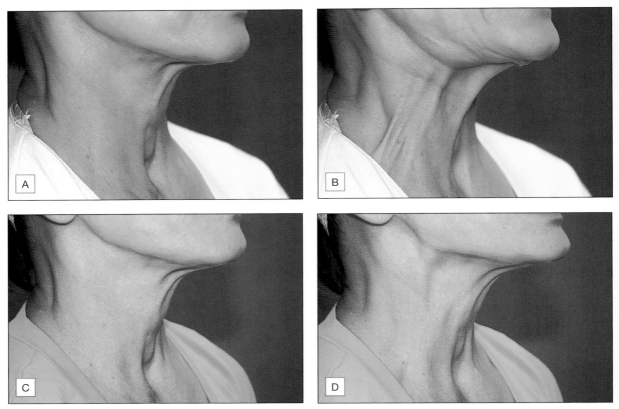

Fig. 7.8 (**A**) Neck at rest before treatment, (**B**) neck contracted before treatment, (**C**) neck at rest after treatment, (**D**) neck contracted after treatment

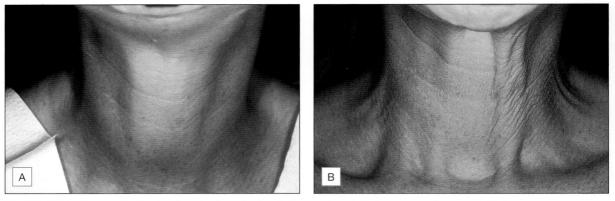

Fig. 7.9 (**A**) Neck at rest before treatment, (**B**) neck at rest after treatment. Note decreased submental fullness

the supine position. Transient headaches have also been noted. For the novice injector, the prudent course may be to start with lower doses and retreat as needed.

Summary

Botulinum toxin injections serve an excellent complementary role in esthetic neck rejuvenation. Patients with mild to moderate neck degenerative changes respond well to treatment. The prior surgical patient or the patient not desirous of an invasive procedure also do well.

Further Reading

Becker-Wegerich PM, Rauch L, Ruzicka T 2002 Botulinum toxin A: successful décolleté rejuvenation. Dermatologic Surgery 28:168–171

Brandt FS, Bellman B 1998 Cosmetic use of botulinum A exotoxin for the aging neck. Dermatologic Surgery 24:1232–1234

Brandt FS, Boker A 2003 Botulinum toxin for rejuvenation of the neck. Clinics in Dermatology 21:513–520

Carruthers J, Carruthers A 2003 Aesthetic botulinum A toxin in the mid and lower face and neck. Dermatologic Surgery 29:468–476

Clarke MSF, Feeback D 1996 Mechanical load induces sarcoplasmic wounding and FGF release in differentiated skeletal muscle cultures. FASEB Journal 10:502–509

Gardetto A, Dabernig J, Rainer C, Piegger J, Piza-Katzer H, Fritsche H 2003 Does a superficial musculoaponeurotic system exist in the face and neck? An anatomical study by the tissue plastination technique. Plastic and Reconstructive Surgery 111:664–672

Goldman MP, Weiss RA 2001 Treatment of poikiloderma of Civatte on the neck with an intense pulsed light source. Plastic and Reconstructive Surgery 107:1376–1381

Hoefflin SM 1996 The platysma aponeurosis. Plastic and Reconstructive Surgery 97:1080

Horn TD 1990 Non-inflammatory disorders of the skin. In: Farmer ER, Hood AF (eds) Pathology of the skin. Appleton & Lange, Norwalk CT, pp. 405

Jacob CI, Kaminer MS 2002 The corset platysma repair: a technique revisited. Dermatologic Surgery 28:257–262

Jacob CI, Berkes BJ, Kaminer MS 2000 Liposuction and surgical recontouring of the neck: a retrospective analysis. Dermatologic Surgery 26:625–632

Krutmann J 2000 Ultraviolet A radiation-induced biologic effects in human skin: relevance for photoaging and photodermatosis. Journal of Dermatological Science S1:S22–26

Matarasso A, Matarasso S, Brandt FS, Bellman B 1999 Botulinum A exotoxin for the management of platysma bands. Plastic and Reconstructive Surgery 103:645–652

Mendelson BC 2001 Surgery of the superficial musculoaponeurotic system: principles of release, vectors, and fixation. Plastic and Reconstructive Surgery 107:1545–1552

Rodriquez AA, Bilkey WJ, Agre JC 1992 Therapeutic exercise in chronic neck and back pain. Archives of Physical Medicine and Rehabilitation 73:870–875

Sterodimas A, Nicolaou M, Paes TRF 2003 Successful use of botulinum toxin A for the treatment of neck and anterior chest wall flushing. Clinics in Experimental Dermatology 28:592–594

Stone J, Brannon T, Haddad F, et al 1996 Adaptive responses of hyper-trophying skeletal muscle to endurance training. Journal of Applied Physiology 81:665–672

Uitto J 1986 Connective tissue biochemistry of the aging dermis: age-related alterations in collagen and elastin. Dermatology Clinics 4:433–446

Vistnes LM, Souther SG 1979 The anatomical basis for common cosmetic anterior neck deformities. Annals of Plastic Surgery 2:381–388

Wheeland RG, Applebaum J 1990 Flashlamp-pumped pulsed dye laser for poikiloderma of Civatte. Journal of Dermatologic Surgery 16:12–16

Yang S, Alnaqeeb M, Simpson H, Goldspink G 1997 Changes in muscle fibre type, muscle mass and IGF-I gene expression in rabbit skeletal muscle endurance training. Journal of Anatomy 190:613–622

Adjunctive Treatment

8

Jeffrey T. S. Hsu, Jean Carruthers

Introduction

> To me, fair Friend, you never can be old,
> For as you were when first your eye I eyed
> Such seems your beauty still...
> — *William Shakespeare*

Although man sees beauty in those dearest to him, regardless of their age, he is often much less forgiving for strangers when their youthful façade fades. Thus there are innumerable methods of rejuvenating the aging face. Without a doubt, one of the most powerful agents is botulinum exotoxin A (BTX-A). For years, following the discovery of the cosmetic benefit of BTX-A, it was compared to other tools of facial rejuvenation. With further understanding of the different modalities, the treatment paradigm has shifted from viewing them as competing to accepting them as complementary technologies. Surgical intervention addresses the gravity-induced changes and eliminates redundant tissue; soft tissue-augmenting agents refortify lost soft tissue and improve contours; energy-based devices induce dermal collagen remodeling and improve epidermal and superficial photodamage; and chemo-denervation by BTX-A reduces the underlying dynamic muscular causation of superficial and deep rhytides. It now makes perfect sense to combine two or more modalities to achieve the optimal cosmetic improvement (Box 8.1).

In general, BTX-A serves to enhance and facilitate other interventions. By diminishing the constant expressive muscle action, BTX-A facilitates the manipulation of the tissues during surgery, prevents or slows the return of the wrinkles caused by muscle action, and allows better healing by reducing the tension exerted on the wound by the underlying muscles. In addition it may have previously undescribed effects on collagen remodeling, pigment accumulation, and vascular tone.

Patient selection

BTX-A is a remarkably safe therapeutic agent. However, certain contraindications do apply (Box 8.2). To prevent bruising, sufficient washout from non-steroidal anti-inflammatory medications, vitamin E, anticoagulants, and aspirin is advised. See Chapter 12 for further discussion of contraindications.

Adjunctive Treatment with Tissue Augmentation

One of the most useful adjunctive applications of BTX-A is the enhancement of the aesthetic effect

---

Adjunctive use of BTX-A

Tissue augmentation
Energy-based devices
Ablative lasers
Nonablative lasers
Radiofrequency
Surgery
Brow lift
Blepharoplasty
Facelift
Wound healing

Box 8.1 Adjunctive use of BTX-A

Contraindications to BTX-A

Neuromuscular disease
Pregnancy
Breastfeeding
Active infection
Allergy to constituents of BTX-A injection
Concurrent use of aminoglycoside

Box 8.2 Contraindications to BTX-A

Tissue augmentation agents
Collagens: Bovine and bioengineered human
Hyaluronic acid
Autologous fat
Silicone
Polymethylmethacrylate (PMMA)
Hydroxyapatite
Polylactic acid
Polyacrylamide
Polytetrafluoroethylene (PTFE)

Box 8.3 Tissue augmentation agents

and duration of soft tissue augmentation. BTX-A can be administered to the desired area approximately 1 week prior to tissue augmentation. The injection of biodegradable dermal filler, subdermal fat, silicone, or surgical implantation then takes place in an area of softened muscular activity. The BTX-A pretreatment serves several purposes. It reduces the dynamic component of the target rhytides, which may allow a more accurate estimation of the volume of filler needed. This prevents overcorrection that could possibly occur when the physician overcompensates for the dynamic component and allows more accurate placement. This is especially critical when using more permanent substances. Second, it may increase the longevity of the implant by decreasing the chronic mechanical microtrauma and inflammation of muscular activity. Third, it helps to maintain the desired position of the implant by reducing microextrusion caused by repetitive motion after injection.

A common application of this synergy is at the glabella, where one weakens the medial brow depressors prior to injection of dermal fillers. A recent study compared the results of treating deep glabellar lines with hyaluronic acid (Restylane, Q-Med AB, Uppsala, Sweden) alone or in combination with BTX-A. The effects of the filler alone lasted an average of 18 weeks, but up to 32 weeks for the group that underwent the combination treatment. This synergy is also seen with the combination of BTX-A weakening of the orbicularis oris muscle and the soft tissue augmentation of the lips and the vermilion borders. The dosages of BTX-A in these adjunctive treatments are similar to those used as primary treatment. BTX-A is compatible with most augmentation agents used in North America (Box 8.3).

Not only is the effective in-tissue duration of the filler lengthened, but the overall cosmetic outcome is enhanced by this combination intervention. While mild to moderate glabellar lines will respond to either BTX-A or fillers, patients who have very deep vertical glabellar grooves may continue to have these lines at rest even after chemodenervation of the underlying muscles. In these cases, BTX-A will address the muscular cause of the rhytides, while dermal support with tissue augmentation will alleviate the residual dermal grooving. These observations have been documented in several studies, which highlight the trend for older subjects who have deeper static lines to require this combination treatment.

Adjunctive Treatment with Energy-Based Devices

Overview

In recent years, lasers have become an indispensable part of the armamentarium in combating photoaging for the cosmetic surgeon. The newest development also includes broadband light and radiofrequency devices. The concomitant use of these devices and BTX-A has led to surprising observations. The lessons learned from these anecdotal experiences are now studied and refined.

Ablative lasers

Ablative laser resurfacing with either carbon dioxide (CO_2) laser or erbium:yttrium aluminum garnet (Er:YAG) laser has shown dramatic facial rejuvenation unmatched by any other treatments (Fig. 8.1). Because these lasers address static wrinkle and BTX-A addresses dynamic wrinkles, the synergy is intuitive. Without concurrent BTX-A use, recurrent dynamic rhytides within 6–12 months are commonplace in the lower eyelid, lateral canthus, and perioral regions as a consequence of continued facial expressivity after resurfacing. In certain cases, the recurrent rhytides can appear even more noticeable than before the resurfacing (Figs 8.2A & 8.2B). Pretreatment with BTX-A diminishes the hyperfunctional rhytides during the postoperative period and allows for healing and remodeling undisturbed by underlying muscle activity. This appears to produce more long-lived reduction of the rhytides. One author (JC) first reported, in a prospective clinical

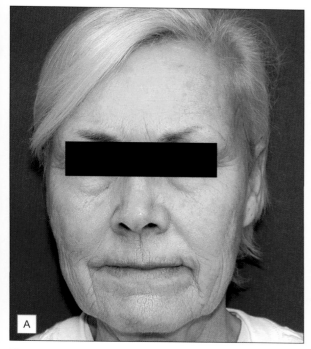 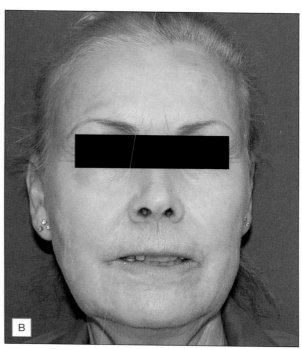

Fig. 8.1 (A, B) Rejuvenation of the photoaged face with CO2 laser

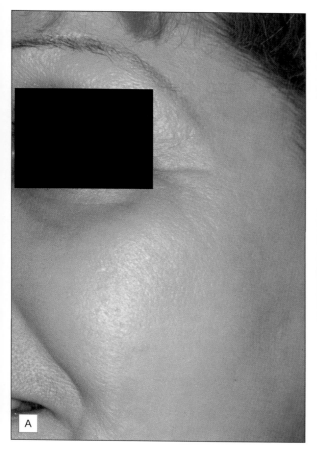 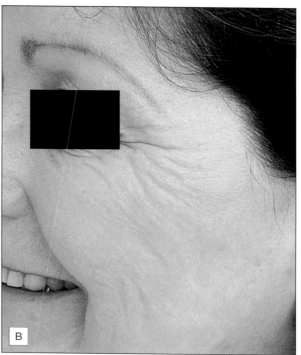

Fig. 8.2 (A, B) Periocular folds became more noticeable after CO2 laser resurfacing due to enhanced thickness of the dermal collagen. BTXA injection masks this change and improves the cosmetic effect of the LSR

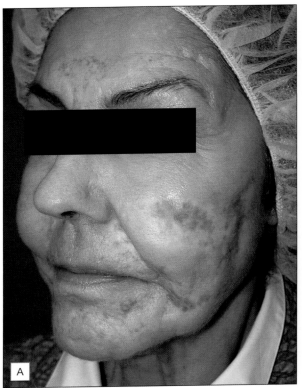 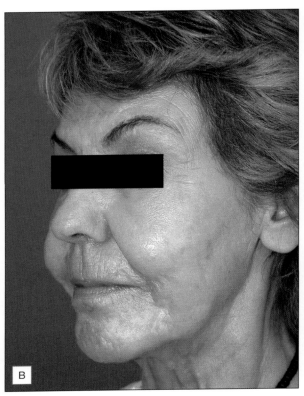

Fig. 8.3 Treatment with intense pulsed light and levulan (α aminolevulinic) following previous treatment with intense pulsed light alone

study, better aesthetic result when combining BTX-A and resurfacing to the periocular area. In a later series of 53 volunteers, those who received BTX-A in the perioperative period had 21% better outcome than those who underwent laser resurfacing alone. Another report confirmed the finding with a study showing enhanced and more prolonged correction of forehead, glabellar, and lateral canthal rhytides over a 9-month period when combining CO_2 laser resurfacing with BTX-A.

This combination is applicable to other areas as well. Laser resurfacing can soften the vertical perioral rhytides ('lipstick lines') and the marionette lines. To complement the effect, BTX-A can soften the depressive pull on the lip corners ('mouth frown') caused by overactive depressor anguli oris muscles and can contribute to the formation of the marionette lines. BTX-A to the orbicularis oris helps to diminish the deep vertical lines caused by the lip sphincter. Either of these treatments must be administered with care to avoid interference with function of the lips and mouth. With proper dosage

and technique, normal speech, whistling, or mastication is unaffected. When full face resurfacing is considered, the laser surgeon may also consider BTX-A chemodenervation of the frontalis, the glabella, and orbicularis oculi and, in some subjects, the zygomaticus complex to enhance the softening of the forehead, periocular rhytides, and nasolabial folds, respectively.

Nonablative light sources

To avoid the recovery time and the risk associated with ablative laser resurfacing, patients and physician now look to nonablative rejuvenation technologies to reverse photoaging. One of the most successful treatment options is the intense pulsed light (IPL), a noninvasive, nonablative broadband light source (Fig. 8.3). Since the introduction of the first commercial IPL system in 1994, refinement of this technology has made it one of the most versatile tools in treating the aging skin. Unlike lasers, IPL is a noncollimated, noncoherent light source. It emits a continuous spectrum that ranges from 500 to 1200 nm, the actual wavelengths used depending on the use of appropriate filters. As with true lasers, the efficacy of IPL in treatment of vascular and pigmented lesions is based on selective destruction of target chromophores by particular wavelengths and pulse durations.. In contrast to CO2 or Er:YAG lasers, the light bypasses the superficial epidermis and targets the underlying melanocytes and dermis, including the microvasculature and melanin components. The pulse duration can range widely from 0.5 to over 20 ms, and pulses can be delivered singly or one following the other (double pulsing) or three in a row (triple pulsing), with variable delay between the pulses. The epidermis can be cooled by applying a thick layer of cold gel, or by integrated cooling on the IPL crystal. Studies have shown that IPL devices are effective for reduction of both lentigenes and vascular lesions, such as telangiectasias, port-wine stains, and poikiloderma.

Along with improvement in red color tone, vessels, dyspigmentation and lentigenes, clinical studies have shown improvements in skin texture, pore size, and fine wrinkles. This is thought to occur through three mechanisms:

- Physical displacement of actinically damaged dermis;
- General dermal injury that leads to collagen reorganization as well as neocollagenesis through fibroblast activation;
- Selective injury to the microvasculature of the papillary dermis that leads to cytokine release, initiating the dermal remodeling cascade.

To our knowledge, the author (JC) and colleagues conducted the only prospective randomized study to explore the effect of BTX-A in combination with IPL. Comparing volunteers receiving only IPL (Quantum SR, Lumenis) treatment to the periorbital area, with those that underwent both BTX-A and IPL, at 6-month evaluation, there was a 15% improvement in overall aesthetic benefit in the latter. Remarkably, the overall improvement in wrinkling, texture, and blemishes in the combined treatment group exceeded those of the IPL-only group more than 6 months after the BTX-A injection, far longer than the expected duration of its direct effect.

Furthermore, the investigators noted improvement in not only texture and wrinkles with the combination treatment, but also vascular and pigmentary lesions as well. The exact mechanism is unknown, but the improvement in telangiectasias underscores the ability of BTX-A to regulate blood vessel constriction, a function that is just beginning to be explored. The recent discovery that BTX-A can treat persistent facial flushing further strengthens this relationship.

It is thought that, at least in part, this enhancement comes from the denervating effect of BTX-A, which prevents the active muscular disturbance of newly deposited dermal collagen. The same mechanism is believed to be the basis of enhancement of nonablative lasers by BTX-A. Several lasers have been developed with the aim of stimulating new collagen growth and improving texture without the prolonged healing and side effects of the resurfacing lasers. Just like IPL, the nonablative lasers are attractive to physicians and patients alike because of the minimal risk and inconvenience. Several infrared lasers, including Nd:YAG laser (1320 nm), diode laser (1450 nm), and Er:Glass laser (1540 nm), deliver thermal injury to the dermis while simultaneously cooling and protecting the epidermis. The thermal injury to the dermis initiates fibroblastic proliferation and upregulation of collagen I expression. Weeks to months after a series of treatments, increased collagen may be observed histologically in the dermis. Instead of causing nonspecific thermal damage to the dermis, vascular lasers, such as KTP laser (532 nm), pulsed dye laser (585, 595 nm), and Nd:YAG laser (1064 nm) induce nonablative remodeling by stimulating the release of inflammatory mediators from vascular endothelial cells, ultimately leading to the production of new dermal collagen by fibroblasts. BTX-A inhibits the underlying muscles from molding the newly formed collagen fibers into nonlinear form.

Nonablative radiofrequency nonsurgical collagen-tightening devices

An energy-based device is quickly gaining popularity in the treatment of photoaging. ThermaCool TC System (Thermage, Hayward, CA) delivers volumetric and uniform heating to the deep dermis via a unique form of radiofrequency (RF) energy, ultimately tightening the skin. Unlike lasers, which target specific chromophores on the principle of selective photothermolysis, RF generates heat based on tissue's natural resistance to the movement of electrons within an RF field. Once the energy is delivered to the tissue, a dual effect is observed. Primary collagen contraction, similar to that seen with ablative CO_2 laser resurfacing, is postulated as a short-term mechanism of action. Secondary collagen synthesis in response to thermal injury is predicted over a longer time period. Studies have documented that thermally modified tissues undergo a remodeling process characterized by fibroplasia and increased collagen deposition. This RF-based skin tightening has been applied to the forehead to achieve nonsurgical browlift, and to the cheeks and jawline for nonsurgical facelift. Although no controlled studies are available, BTX-A has already been used to enhance the results of this device. The immobilization of the musculature, especially of the brow depressors, should augment the elevation of the brows and prolong the duration of the result. Additionally, just as in nonablative lasers, BTX-A inhibits the underlying muscles from molding the newly formed collagen into more wrinkles.

Adjunctive Treatment with Surgery

Overview

Surgical approaches to the face and neck can offer stunning improvement, but results can be short-lived. Surgical procedures that yield suboptimal results can be attributed to the failure to understand the causative roles that dynamic musculature plays in the creation of soft tissue changes. Surgeons now realize that, although surgery may remove skin redundancy, they do not address the activity of mimetic muscles, which over time can reverse the correction.

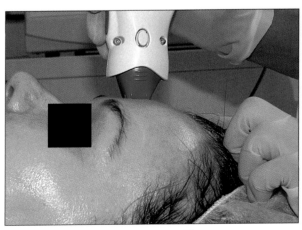

Fig. 8.4 Treatment with ThermaCool TC system

Likewise, muscle activity partially contributes to the malpositioning of certain facial features, such as brow ptosis. Therefore, in repositioning these features, one must address the role of the related muscle in the cause of the problem and in the recovery process. Chemodenervation with BTX-A is now a key adjunct to several aesthetic surgery interventions.

Brow lift

Ptosis of the brow is the result of photodamage and the habitual and repetitive use of the brows in everyday expressions. The depressed brow position confers projected emotional content of fatigue, frustration, and anger, however unintended. Mild brow ptosis (<2 mm) can be corrected with BTX-A alone (Figs 8.4, 8.5A & 8.5B). Chemical brow lift through BTX-A was discovered serendipitously from treatment of glabellar frown lines, when it became apparent that the medial brows were elevated as well.

While there are four muscles that supply the downward vector force, only one muscle, the frontalis, supplies the upward vector. By weakening all four

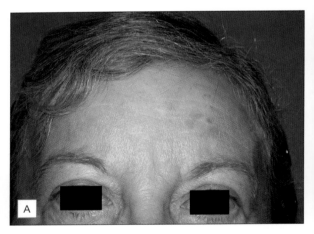

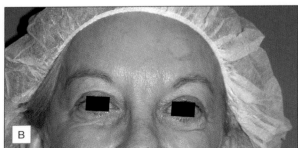

Fig. 8.5 (A, B) Mild brow ptosis corrected with BTX-A alone

muscles, the procerus, the corrugator, the depressor supercilii, and the orbicularis oculi, one can achieve 1–2 mm brow lift consistently. Although at times considered to be a part of the corrugator or the orbicularis oculi, a study described the depressor supercilii as a distinct muscle originating from the nasal process of the frontal bone and inserting into the skin just inferior to the medial head of the eyebrow. It has also been shown that denervation of this muscle can lead to marked elevation of the medial brow.

In treatment of the brow depressors, it is important to avoid over-affecting the frontalis, as this would have the opposite effect of lowering the brows. The inferior portion of the frontalis muscle interdigitates with the brow depressors, and thus can be affected when the depressors are injected. Because the bulk of the frontalis is superior to the brows, injecting at a point immediately below a line joining the eyebrows should minimize ptosis. Furthermore, using a high toxin concentration of 1 u/0.01 cc also helps to limit diffusion from the point of injection.

In addition to location and concentration, the dosage is also important. Initial experiences with BTX-A brow lift showed that excessive treatment of the glabella with large doses (up to 25 u for women and up to 35 u for men) often paralyzed not just the depressors, but the frontalis as well. It was found that lower doses (7–10 u) paradoxically raised the medial brows more consistently. The lower doses also permitted voluntary frowning and other natural facial expressions. The lateral brows are elevated by injection into the supralateral eyebrow above the lateral canthus. However, a recent dose-ranging study by the author (JC) and colleagues has shown a small and transient brow ptosis with smaller doses. This compares with approximately a 1mm brow lift in women with doses of 20–40 u (unpublished data). The authors surmise that, as the larger doses allowed enough diffusion to weaken the medial frontalis, the result was that the body compensates by increasing innervation to the entire frontalis muscle. Because the lateral fibers are less affected, they provide lift to the lateral brows. For further discussion of this subject see Chapter 4.

For moderate to severe brow ptosis (3–10 mm), the surgical approach is usually needed. Endoscopic brow lifting has gained wide acceptance over the classic bicoronal lift due to the less invasive nature of the newer procedure. Only a few incisions are made behind the post-trichal scalp so that the resulting scars will be less visible. Through endoscopy, the fibrous connections of the brow to the orbital margins are dissected and the brow depressor muscles are extirpated. BTX-A complements brow lift operations in several ways. Brow lifts may have unpredictable outcome depending on the postsurgical healing. Stabilization of the brow musculature is essential as periosteal refixation requires approximately 12 weeks. During this healing period, surgeons need to fix the patients' brows in elevated positions to prevent a quick descent. BTX-A provides the perfect tool to chemically maintain the brows in elevated positions by weakening the inferior vector force. Furthermore, surgical excision of the depressor fibers may lead to uneven regrowth of the muscles. Pretreatment with BTX-A may circumvent this possible complication.

Postoperatively, the brow elevations provided by endoscopic brow lifts are often compromised within 6 months, in as many as 40% of cases. BTX-A in these cases can extend the duration of lift. BTX-A can also be used to correct eyebrow asymmetry after brow lift surgery (Figs 8.6A & 8.6B). One could chemodenervate the frontalis muscle above the higher brow and/or the depressor muscles of the lower brow to achieve even brow height, although elevation of the lower brow is often the most appropriate aesthetic choice.

Surgeons who recognize the utility of BTX-A not only use it as an adjunctive treatment to browlift, but may even choose BTX-A over surgery in some cases. Since its introduction in 1992, endoscopic brow lift has gained wide recognition as a novel technique to correct brow ptosis in a minimally invasive manner with fewer complications than the classic coronal brow lift method. However, the number of endoscopic brow lift procedures performed has declined by as much as 70% in certain institutions. Several factors account for the decline in the popularity of this procedure. Not only are the long-term results disappointing to some surgeons, the observed postsurgical complications included alopecia, hairline changes, brow asymmetry, paresthesia, frontal branch nerve paralysis, and scalp dysesthesia. These complications were similar to those resulting from open brow lifts. Many surgeons have observed that chemodenervation from BTX-A results in a brow lift that approaches endoscopic lift in magnitude without having to subject the patient to invasive surgery with the risk for complications.

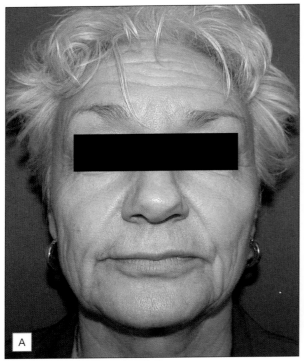
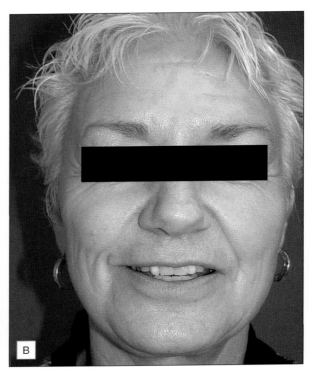

Fig. 8.6 Uneven brow height can be reset preoperatively with Botox so that the appropriate surgical plan for the aesthetic blepharoplasty can be followed

Blepharoplasty

Pretreatment with BTX-A can prevent complications from upper eyelid blepharoplasty. Many blepharoplasty candidates have one brow slightly lower than the other, often the side on which they sleep (Fig. 8.7). The surgeon may remove more skin on this side unknowingly, resulting in a hostile or worried expression. A BTX-A lift as described in the previous section creates brows of equal height prior to the surgery (Fig. 8.7). This could help the surgeon properly plan the operation. The pretreatment of the crow's feet permits the surgeon to hide the incision line within the bony orbital margin without feeling the need to address the crow's feet surgically. This limits the scope of the surgery and gives a superior aesthetic result. The surgeon may also explain the asymmetry to the patient and recommend concurrent transblepharoplasty superolateral browplexy to the frontal periosteum or other brow lifting procedure before the blepharoplasty.

For the lower blepharoplasty, BTX-A serves to enhance wound healing. The results of the surgery are often compromised by the repetitive muscular

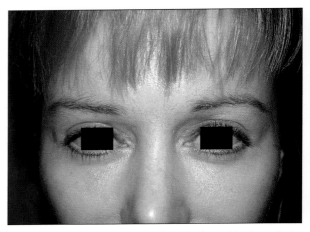

Fig. 8.7 Uneven brow height is found prior to blepharoplasty in approximately 80% of adult female candidates

actions that distort the outcome. For example, tarsal strip procedure for the treatment of ectropion is often plagued by the dehiscence of the temporal repair of the distal tarsus to the lateral canthal tendon. Prior to the operation, 5 u of BTX-A to the lateral orbicularis to minimize the pulling action tend to

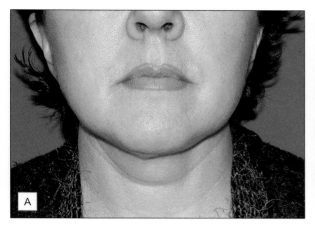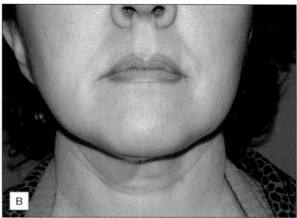

Fig. 8.8 Preoperative Botox into the face and neck depressor muscle, the platysma, can prevent unwanted tension on the face lift incision and allow optimal wound healing

reduce the rate of dehiscence and treat the lateral canthal rhytides (crow's feet) at the same time

A recent investigation in the injection of BTX-A into orbicularis muscles under direct surgical vision during blepharoplasty revealed paralysis for up to 12 months, confirmed by electromyographic studies, a duration much longer than transcutaneous injections. Furthermore, the muscle paralysis started within 24 hours, faster than the usual 3–5 days observed with transcutaneous injections. Although these observations are controversial and may be specific to the dose and the technique, they hint at the synergy between chemodenervation and surgery at a molecular level, although the mechanisms are unclear. However, some investigators call into question the safety of intraoperative injections. For example, the toxin may migrate inadvertently through disrupted tissue planes into undesired areas. Furthermore, neutralizing antibodies to BTX-A has been rare, and limited to frequent injections in doses larger than 100 u during transcutaneous injections and with the Allergan BTX-A original pre-1997 formulation. There is the theoretical possibility that the trauma of surgery and subsequent inflammatory response may potentiate the immune response responsible for development of IgG-neutralizing antibodies to BTX-A. However, there has been no report of neutralizing antibodies since BTX-A was reformulated into its present low protein form by Allergan in 1997. The authors also prefer pretreatment over intraoperative treatment to relax the muscles prior to surgery, allowing for more accurate estimation of the amount the tissue to be resected.

Facelift

Facelift, necklift, and platysma repair surgeries involve the imbrication of the superficial musculoaponeurotic system and the plication of the platysma muscle. The activity of the platysma pulls the skin downward and can reverse the effect of the procedures over time. Injection of the platysma before and after the procedures may enhance the longevity of the outcome (Fig. 8.8). Dysphagia and weakness of neck flexion is unlikely when the dose is limited to 30–40 u.

BTX-A is useful in resolving postfacelift synkinesis seen in peripheral damage to the buccal branch of the facial nerve. This results in the unintentional sneer due to the activation of the levator labii superioris or zygomaticus muscle whenever the patient blinks. The levator labii superioris may be injected with 1 or 2 u to diminish this complication. Likewise, the neck liposuction that often accompanies facelifts and platysma repairs can rarely injure the marginal mandibular nerve that controls the depressors of the lower lip. BTX-A administered to the contralateral side may maintain the symmetry of the mouth, allowing symmetry to be re-established while the contralateral marginal mandibular nerve recovers.

Wound healing

The importance of proper planning and orientation of the surgical wound cannot be overstated. However, at times, especially in repair of traumatic wounds, muscular action impedes the healing of wounds oriented unfavorably to the relaxed tension line. A study demonstrated the value in pretreating the underlying musculature with BTX-A. Immobilization of the muscles promoted healing of the wound. The repetitive microtrauma caused by displacement of the injured tissue prolongs the inflammatory response, leading to a more exuberant scar formation. BTX-A minimizes the repetitive tension on the wound edge, resulting in a cosmetically superior scar. Furthermore, the lack of disruptive tension on the wound allows the surgeon to use finer sutures to achieve better cosmesis.

Conclusion

The cosmetic use of BTX-A continues to expand as physicians now regard it as a helpful adjunct with a number of cosmetic procedures. While physicians who offer BTX-A and other methods of rejuvenations may have already discovered this synergy through experience and intuition, few have systematically categorized the many combinations. We eagerly await more discoveries of adjunctive uses of BTX-A and more controlled studies to refine the techniques and to ensure the biocompatibility and the patient satisfaction of the various combinations.

Further Reading

Anderson RR. Laser tissue interactions in dermatology. In: Arndt KA, Dover JS, eds. Lasers in Cutaneous and Aesthetic Surgery. Lippincott-Raven, Philadelphia, 1997:25.

Carruthers J, Carruthers A. Combining botulinum toxin injection and laser for facial rhytides. In: Coleman WP; Lawrence N, eds. Skin Resurfacing. Williams and Wilkins, Baltimore, MD, 1998:235–243.

Carruthers J, Carruthers A. The adjunctive usage of botulinum toxin. Dermatological Surgery 1998;24:1244–1247.

Carruthers J, Carruthers A. A prospective, randomized, parallel group study analyzing the effect of BTX-A (BOTOX) and nonanimal sourced hyaluronic acid (NASHA, Restylane) in combination compared with NASHA (Restylane) alone in severe glabellar rhytides in adult female subjects: treatment of severe glabellar rhytides with a hyaluronic acid derivative compared with the derivative and BTX-A. Dermatological Surgery 2003;29:802–809.

Carruthers J, Carruthers A, Zelichowska A. The power of combined therapies: botox and ablative facial laser resurfacing. American Journal of Cosmetic Surgery 2000;17:129–131.

Carruthers JA, Weiss R, Narurkar V, Flynn TC. Intense pulsed light and botulinum toxin type A for the aging face. Cosmetic Dermatology 2003b;16(11, Supp 5): 2–16.

Chen TH, Wei FC 1997 Evolution of the vertical reduction mammaplasty: the S approach. Aesthetic Plastic Surgery 21(2):97–104.

Cook BE Jr, Lucarelli MJ, Lemke BN 2001 Depressor supercilii muscle: anatomy, histology, and cosmetic implications. Ophthalmic Plastic and Reconstructive Surgery 17(6):404–411.

Fagien S, Brandt FS. Primary and adjunctive use of botulinum toxin type A (Botox) in facial aesthetic surgery: beyond the glabella. Clinics in Plastic Surgery 2001;28(1):127–148.

Frankel AS, Kamer FM. Chemical browlift. Archives in Otological Head and Neck Surgery 1998;124:321–323.

Gassner HG, Sherris DA, Otley CC. Treatment of facial wounds with botulinum toxin A improves cosmetic outcome in primates. Plastic and Reconstructive Surgery 2000;105(6):1948–1953; discussion 1954–1955.

Guerrissi JO. Intraoperative injection of botulinum toxin A into the orbicularis oculi muscle for the treatment of crow's feet. Plastic and Reconstructive Surgery 2003;112(5 Suppl):161S–163S.

Hsu TS, Alam M, Dover JS. Laser and light based treatment of the aging skin. In: Rigel DS, Weiss RA, Lim HW, Dover JS, eds. Photoaging. Marcel Dekker, New York, 2004:141–181.

Huilgol S. Carruthers JA, Carruthers JDA. Raising eyebrows with botulinum toxin. Dermatological Surgery 1999;25:373–376.

Jacob CI, Berkes BJ, Kaminer MS. Liposuction and surgical recontouring of the neck: a retrospective analysis. Dermatological Surgery 2000;26(7):625–632.

Lovice D. Botulinum toxin use in facial plastic surgery. Otolaryngological Clinics in North America 2002;35(1):171–186.

Mandeville JT, Rubin PA. Injectable agents for facial rejuvenation: botulinum toxin and dermal filling agents. International Ophthalmological Clinics 2004;44(1):189–212.

Weiss RA, Weiss MA, Beasley KL. Rejuvenation of photoaged skin: 5-year results with intense pulsed light of the face, neck, and chest. Dermatological Surgery 2002;28(12):1115–1119.

West TB, Alster TS. Effect of botulinum toxin type A on movement-associated rhytides following CO2 laser resurfacing. Dermatological Surgery 1999;25(4):259–261.

Worcester S. Use botox before and after laser facial resurfacing. Skin and Allergy News 2000;31:6.

Yuraitis M, Jacob CI. Botulinum toxin for the treatment of facial flushing. Dermatological Surgery 2004;30(1):102–104.

Management of Hyperhidrosis

9

Aamir Haider, Nowell Solish, Nicholas J. Lowe

Introduction

Hyperhidrosis is characterized by sweating in excess of the physiologic amount necessary to maintain thermal homeostasis. For those affected, this condition is extremely debilitating with significant impairment in activities of daily living, social interaction, and occupational activities. Hyperhidrosis is divided into primary or idiopathic hyperhidrosis and secondary due to a variety of causes. This classification is further categorized as generalized or focal with respect to its clinical presentation. Primary or idiopathic hyperhidrosis is usually focal and limited to the axillae, palms and soles, and face. Secondary hyperhidrosis can be focal or generalized, affecting the entire body. The focus of this chapter is on the diagnosis and management of hyperhidrosis, with a focus on primary focal idiopathic hyperhidrosis. With a reported prevalence of 2.8% of the population, and associated significant psychosocial morbidity, it is imperative that physicians recognize this disease entity and understand the various treatment modalities that are available. Treatment strategies for hyperhidrosis include topical, oral, surgical, and nonsurgical treatments. These treatment modalities differ with respect to their therapeutic efficacy, duration of effect, side effects, as well as cost of therapy.

Problem being treated

A standard definition of excessive sweating has not yet been established. Quantification of sweat production in studies has ranged from normal being defined as less than $1 \, mL/m^2/min$ to the production of less than 100 mg of sweat in one axilla within 5 min, or less than 50 mg within 1 min. The fundamental criticism of these measurement parameters is the fact that they fail to take into account surface area. As a consequence, smaller people may end up falling below this quantitative definition, despite excessive and debilitating sweating. For practical purposes, any degree of sweating that interferes with activities of daily living can be viewed as hyperhidrosis.

Clinical presentation

Symptoms of excessive sweating generally begin in adolescence but may present even earlier. In a study of Taiwanese patients with palmar hyperhidrosis, 75% had a childhood onset, with the rest presenting in puberty. A recent survey of a nationally representative sample of 150 000 households in the USA revealed an average age of onset of 25. The average age of onset for axillary hyperhidrosis was 19 years, and 13 years for palmar hyperhidrosis. In some patients, sweat production can be as high as 40 times the normal rate of $1 \, mL/m^2/min$, as defined in one study. Patients generally present with sweating of one or more anatomic regions such as axillae, palms, soles, or face. The US survey revealed that 51% of patients with hyperhidrosis had axillary involvement alone or in combination with another site, and 9.5% reported axillary involvement alone. Palmar hyperhidrosis alone or in combination with another site was reported in 25% of patients, and only 1% reported palmar hyperhidrosis alone. Plantar hyperhidrosis alone or in combination with another site was reported in 30% of patients. Facial hyperhidrosis was reported in 10% of patients.

Because there is no well established definition of hyperhidrosis, it is reasonable to diagnose this condition in people who report excessive sweating that interferes with activities of daily living. A high index of suspicion is critical to diagnose this condition, as a significant proportion of patients do not realize that they have a medical issue or feel too embarrassed to seek help. Canadian data reported that 75% of men and 64% of women with hyperhidrosis had not consulted their physician about the condition.

An essential component of the clinical assessment of patients with hyperhidrosis is the realization of the significant impact of this condition on the quality of life of patients. A recent survey in the USA reported that 34–47% of patients felt that their sweating had a moderate to severe effect on limitations at work, meeting people, and in romantic or intimate situations. This study also reported that 32% of patients with axillary hyperhidrosis indicated that their sweating is barely tolerable or intolerable, and frequently or always interferes with their daily activities. A reported 35% of patients decreased the amount of time spent in leisure activities. Over 50% of patients with axillary hyperhidrosis in the US survey reported feeling less confident, 34% reported feeling unhappy, 38% reported feeling frustrated with daily activities, and 20% reported feeling depressed.

Hyperhidrosis has a profound impact on social interactions and work-related acitivites. Routine social interactions such as holding hands, shaking hands, or hugging become awkward. Patients report a sense of humiliation and embarrassment associated with soaked or stained clothing as well as perceived odours. Palmar hyperhidrosis can dramatically affect occupational and social activities. Patients report difficulty with holding tools, drawing or writing, and often paper ends up being stained with sweat or smeared ink. Occupations involving contact with paper, metal or electrical equipment were noted in a study to be unattainable for patients with palmar hyperhidrosis. Patients with axillary hyperhidrosis treated with botulinum toxin (BTX) in a large multicenter study were assessed using the Hyperhidrosis Impact Questionnaire. A total of 71% of patients reported being less confident than they would like to be, 49% were unhappy or depressed, 30% were frustrated with daily activities, 25% missed social gatherings with loved ones, 32% felt at least moderately limited with regard to sexual activities, and 81% felt limited with respect to meeting people for the first time. As one would expect, a great deal of time is invested in coping with this problem, with resulting negative consequences both socially and economically.

Pathophysiology of hyperhidrosis

There are approximately 2–4 million sweat glands distributed throughout the skin. The majority, approximately 3 million, are eccrine glands. The remaining are apocrine and apo-eccrine glands.

Eccrine glands, responsible for focal hyperhidrosis, are distributed over almost the entire body surface area, with the most numerous being on the soles of the feet and the forehead, followed by the palms and cheek. The main role of the eccrine glands is a thermoregulatory function, which is also affected by emotional and gustatory stimuli. Histologically, eccrine glands are composed of a secretory coil in the deep dermis and superficial fat, a duct that traverses the dermis and an intraepidermal pore that passes between keratinocytes and opens to the skin surface. Of note is that histological studies have revealed no increase in the number or size of eccrine glands in patients who have hyperhidrosis. The eccrine glands are innervated by sympathetic nerve fibers. These fibers originate in the hypothalamus and descend through the ipsilateral brain stem, forming a synapse with the intermediolateral cell nucleus of the spinal cord. The final innervation of the eccrine sweat glands is with unmyelinated post-ganglionic sympathetic nerve fibers. The primary neurotransmitter released at the periglandular nerve endings is acetylcholine. Periglandular nerve endings also contain catecholamines and neuropeptides; however, their exact role in sweat production is yet to be defined. In light of normal eccrine gland histology in hyperhidrosis, it is believed that hyperhidrosis is due to sympathetic overactivity. Hyperhidrosis may result from a dysfunction of the central sympathetic nervous system that affects the hypothalamic nuclei, prefrontal areas, or their cholinergic connections downstream. The neurogenic overactivity in focal hyperhidrosis may be the result of hyperexcitability of these reflex circuits that are involved in eccrine secretion. There is likely a heritable component to this neurogenic overactivity, as 30–50% of patients have a positive family history.

Apocrine glands are primarily confined to the axillae and urogenital regions. The ratio of apocrine to eccrine sweat glands has been reported as 1:1 in the axilla and 1:10 in other areas. There are also mixed apo-eccrine glands which develop from eccrine-like precursor glands during puberty. The exact roles of apocrine and apo-eccrine glands in hyperhidrosis remains unclear, although in some patients with hyperhidrosis up to 45% of the axillary sweat glands are apo-eccrine glands.

Etiology

Hyperhidrosis is classified as primary or secondary. The clinical presentation is classified as focal or generalized. Primary hyperhidrosis is considered idiopathic and generally presents as focal hyperhidrosis. Focal hyperhidrosis is localized to specific body areas such as the axillae, palms, feet, or face. Secondary hyperhidrosis is most commonly generalized (involves the entire body); however, it can present in a localized, focal pattern. Secondary hyperhidrosis, as the name implies, is due to a variety of secondary causes (Table 9.1) These secondary causes may include underlying medical conditions, drugs, or exaggerated physiological responses to heat, humidity, or exercise.

It is beyond the scope of this chapter comprehensively to review all the causes of secondary hyperhidrosis; however, we mention certain conditions that should be kept in mind as one evaluates a patient. Secondary generalized hyperhidrosis is seen with various medical conditions such as endocrine disorders including thyrotoxicosis, diabetes mellitus, hyperpituitarism, pheochromocytoma, acute and chronic infections, malignancies, and conditions associated with a high sympathetic discharge such as cardiovascular shock, respiratory failure, and alcohol or drug withdrawal. Secondary hyperhidrosis can also present as focal or localized hyperhidrosis. Secondary hyperhidrosis in a focal presentation is most commonly related to neurological injury. Acute spinal cord injury with or without autonomic dysreflexia can present with focal hyperhidrosis of the face or upper trunk, seen months to years after the injury. Post-traumatic syringomyelia following spinal cord injury may also cause focal hyperhidrosis. Cerebrovascular accidents involving hemispheric or medullary infarcts can lead to focal hyperhidrosis on the ipsilateral or contralateral sides, respectively. Other causes of secondary focal hyperhidrosis include

Etiology of hyperhidrosis	
Generalized hyperhidrosis	**Focal hyperhidrosis**

Neurologic
  Parkinson's disease
  Spinal cord injury
  Cerebrovascular accident
	Primary idiopathic
	Axillary
	Palmar
	Plantar
	Facial

Endocrine
  Hyperthyroidism
  Hyperpituitarism
  Diabetes mellitus
  Menopause
  Pregnancy
  Pheochromocytoma
  Carcinoid syndrome
  Acromegaly
	Gustatory sweating (Frey's syndrome)
	
	Associated with neuropathies
	
	Secondary to spinal disease/injury

Infectious	

Cardiovascular
  Shock
  Heart failure	

Respiratory failure	
Drugs	

Toxic
  Alcoholism
  Substance abuse	

Malignancies
  Myeloproliferative disorders
  Hodgkin's disease	

Table 9.1 Etiology of hyperhidrosis

injury to the sympathetic chain due to accessory cervical ribs or an intrathoracic tumor impinging on the sympathetic chain. Frey's syndrome or facial gustatory sweating is also a form of secondary focal hyperhidrosis, due to parotid surgery or trauma. Frey's syndrome is believed to be the result of transection of the postganglionic sympathetic nerve fibers from the otic ganglion that were originally directed to the parotid gland. Following this transection, an aberrant reinnervation of the facial cholinergic sweat glands accounts for the excessive sweating. An awareness of these conditions is helpful in the initial evaluation of a patient with hyperhidrosis. Overall, the most common type of hyperhidrosis remains primary (idiopathic) focal hyperhidrosis, presenting in the axillae, palms, feet, or face.

Patient selection

A recent survey of 150 000 households in the USA revealed that 2.8% of the population or 7.8 million people reported having unusual or excessive sweating. Of those with hyperhidrosis, 62% did not consult a physician for evaluation of their condition. For those with primary focal axillary hyperhidrosis, the numbers are even higher as 61% of women and 73% of men did not consult a physician. Of the 7.8 million people with hyperhidrosis, 2.4 million indicated that their sweating was barely tolerable and frequently interfered with activities of daily living. The prevalence was highest among individuals aged 25–64. No gender differences were noted in prevalence. The average age of onset was 25 years. The average age of onset for axillary hyperhidrosis was 19 years, and 13 years for those with palmar hyperhidrosis. Of note is the fact that other studies have revealed that primary focal hyperhidrosis generally has an onset during childhood or adolescence. A study of 850 patients with axillary, palmar or facial hyperhidrosis revealed that 62% of patients had their symptoms for as long as they could remember, with 33% describing an onset in puberty and 5% with an adult onset. In light of these findings, it would appear that hyperhidrosis is a disease of childhood which appears to peak in early adulthood. Neonatal cases have been described but are not as common. Therefore the early identification and proper management of this debilitating condition is essential to prevent long-term psychosocial morbidity. There is a reported positive family history in 30–50% of patients.

Diagnostic and Treatment Approach

The most common type of hyperhidrosis is primary focal (idiopathic) hyperhidrosis; however, it is critical when evaluating a patient that one is aware of the secondary causes. A thorough history and focused exam will allow one to differentiate primary from secondary hyperhidrosis.

The multispecialty working group on recognition, diagnosis, and treatment of primary focal hyperhidrosis has defined primary focal (idiopathic) hyperhidrosis as focal visible, excessive sweating of at least 6 months' duration without apparent cause with at least two of the following characteristics:

- bilateral and relatively symmetrical
- impairs daily activities
- frequency of at least one episode per week
- age of onset less than 25 years
- positive family history
- cessation of focal sweating during sleep.

Hyperhidrosis associated with symptoms such as fever, night sweats, weight loss, lymphadenopathy, headache or palpitations should alert the physician to evaluate the patient further for possible secondary causes. Therefore, a history focussing on location of excessive sweating, duration of the presentation, associated symptoms or co-morbidities, family history, age of onset, and any specific triggers allows one to differentiate primary from secondary hyperhidrosis.

Once a diagnosis of primary (idiopathic) focal hyperhidrosis is established, the extent of hyperhidrosis can be measured either gravimetrically, as the rate of sweat production (expressed in mg/min), by the iodine starch test, or the ninhydrin test. Gravimetry utilizes a filter paper which is weighed before and after contact with the affected area. Patients are instructed to rest for at least 15 minutes at a room temperature of 21–25 degrees Celsius, before the filter paper is applied to the affected area for 60 seconds and then weighed again. The rate of sweat production in milligrams per minute is then calculated. By gravimetry, axillary hyperhidrosis is defined as > 100 mg/5 min in men and > 50 mg/5 min in women. Palmar hyperhidrosis is defined as > 30–40 mg/min. The starch iodine test is based on the reaction of starch and iodine in the presence of sweat. The area to be tested is dried and iodine solution (1–5%) is applied and after a few seconds starch is sprinkled over this area. The starch and iodine interact in the presence of sweat to develop a

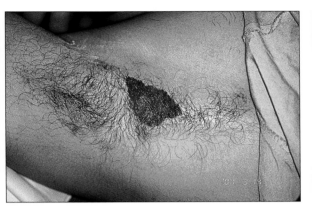

Fig. 9.1 Starch iodine of axillary hyperhidrosis

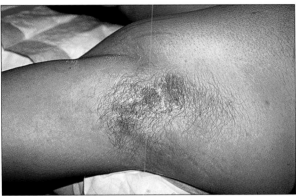

Fig. 9.2 Starch iodine of axilla 2 weeks after treatment with BTX-A

purplish color. This purple area identifies the orifice of the sweat gland. This test allows the qualitative identification of areas of excessive sweating which can be recorded by pictures taken before and after treatment. In order to obtain good results, the authors recommend thorough drying of the area before applying the iodine solution and allowing it to dry for a few seconds before applying the starch. Simple cornstarch can be used and should be applied through a fine dispenser and lightly dusted on the area. This usually will give the most accurate results (Fig. 9.1). Under procedure, the minor starch iodine test is usually photographed before and after treatment in order to demonstrate the objective evidence of improvement. This test will also increase the accuracy of the injection technique (Fig. 9.2).

Finally, the Ninhydrin test is based on the principle that ninhydrin reacts with amino acids in sweat and the resulting impression is visualized using digital analysis of the image produced on paper. This allows quantification of sweat production.

Treatment techniques and strategies

Treatment of hyperhidrosis can be divided into topical, oral, surgical, and nonsurgical treatments. Each of these therapeutic interventions is different with respect to the indications for its use, therapeutic efficacy, duration of action, side effects, and cost of therapy. Treatment of hyperhidrosis needs to be individualized depending on the clinical presentation and a discussion with the patient as to their preferences is critical to ensure reasonable expectations while avoiding unnecessary frustration.

Topical treatments

Topical treatments for hyperhidrosis are characterized by short-term duration of action, with efficacy limited to mild cases of focal hyperhidrosis. Although there are over 90 different compounds available, aluminum chloride hexahydrate is considered the most effective topical agent. Aluminum chloride is available as a 20–25% solution in water or ethanol. The mechanism of action involves a mechanical obstruction of the eccrine sweat gland pore. Long-term use of aluminum chloride products is associated with histological changes such as atrophy of the secretory cells. Prior to application, the skin is dried to avoid irritation, which appears to be the main limiting side effect of this product. The main indication for aluminum chloride is for focal axillary hyperhidrosis; however, it also appears to have short-term efficacy in palmar hyperhidrosis. Other topical products include glycopyrrolate, a topical anticholinergic product available as topical pads for mild cases of hyperhidrosis.

Other topical agents used for focal hyperhidrosis have included glutaraldehyde 10% and formaldehyde; however, the utility of these products is limited due to an enhanced potential for skin irritation and allergic skin sensitization.

Systemic treatments

Systemic anticholinergic treatments are the primary oral agents available for treatment of hyperhidrosis. The main concern with these agents is the fact that, at doses that may reduce hyperhidrosis, the side effects (including dry mouth, blurred vision, constipation, urinary retention, and palpitations) are generally not tolerable. Oral glycopyrrolate at doses of 1 mg two or three times a day is a reasonable initial starting regimen. Other anticholinergic agents have included Amitriptyline.

Benodiazepines such as clonazepam have been reported in cases with a significant emotional component; however, their use has been limited due to the potential for sedation. Other oral agents that have been tried include diltiazem, clonidine, and nonsteroidal anti-inflammatory drugs; however, their efficacy to date has largely been confined to isolated case reports.

Overall, the exact role for oral treatments has not yet been clearly defined in hyperhidrosis. Larger case series or randomized controlled data are needed to determine the true efficacy and role of these agents.

Iontophoresis

Iontophoresis is defined as the introduction of an ionized substance (usually tap water) through intact skin by means of an electrical current. Alternatives to tap water include anticholinergics such as glycopyrrolate or atropine sulfate. This method of treatment is mainly indicated for palmar and plantar hyperhidrosis. The mechanism of action appears to be distal duct blockage. Iontophoresis has several advantages as a means of treatment as there is no systemic use of drugs and patients can utilize this treatment at home. The main disadvantages include the one-off cost, which can range from US\$ 600 to 1000 and the time-consuming frequency of treatments (can be several times a week for 30–40 minutes). Iontophoresis has an efficacy of up to 90% in palmar and plantar hyperhidrosis with multiple treatments. This treatment is generally well tolerated with the potential for mild irritation and dryness. A randomized, controlled double-blind study of iontophoresis in 11 patients with palmar hyperhidrosis and sham treatment of the other hand reported a 38% reduction in sweat production by gravimetry with 10 initial treatments at 4 mA. Maintenance treatments over a 3-month period at 10 mA resulted in an 81% reduction in sweat production.

Iontophoresis is a safe and effective treatment for palmar and plantar hyperhidrosis. The frequency of treatment is generally three to four times a week for approximately 30 minutes. Efficacy has been reported in the range of 80–90% within 3 months; however, long-term maintenance therapy is generally required. The main contraindications for this treatment modality include a pacemaker, orthopedic prosthesis, heart arrhythmias, and pregnancy. Iontophoresis is indicated as a second-line treatment for palmar or plantar hyperhidrosis following topical treatments.

Surgical treatments

Surgical treatments for hyperhidrosis include excision of the axillary vault to remove eccrine glands, curettage or liposuction to remove glandular tissue and, finally, sympathectomy. Appropriate patient selection and detailed patient information is critical in light of the associated postoperative morbidity and complications. Surgical treatment options are generally reserved for patients who fail to respond to all other therapeutic modalities.

Excision of the axillary vault to remove eccrine glands is reported to have an efficacy in the range of 50–90%. Various surgical techniques have been described; however, there are no randomized, controlled trials evaluating this method of treatment. Excision of the axillary vault can be complicated by infection, bleeding, delayed healing, flap necrosis, and significant scarring. Subcutaneous curettage of the axillae was attempted to decrease the postoperative morbidity associated with excisional techniques. Curettage of the axilla is done using a small incision, with a goal to destroy eccrine glandular tissue. Results with this procedure have been mixed as reported attempts at duplicating the initial results have been disappointing, with high relapse rates and poor patient satisfaction. Axillary liposuction has also been advocated in an attempt to destroy and remove glandular tissue, with acceptable efficacy and fewer side effects than traditional techniques. Liposuction tends to cause minimal scarring compared to excision and has a lower risk of bleeding. With all these surgical axillary techniques, the potential for scarring that may subsequently restrict superior arm rotation is present.

Endoscopic thoracic sympathectomy (ETS) destroys the sympathetic ganglia by excision, ablation or clipping. ETS has been performed most frequently for palmar hyperhidrosis and success rates are reported as high as 98%. Several studies validate the efficacy of ETS in palmar and axillary hyperhidrosis. Of note, however, is that long-term outcome studies have reported that patient satisfaction declined over time, with 67% of patients being completely satisfied and 27% partially satisfied after a mean follow-up of 16 years. The main complications with sympathectomy include compensatory sweating, phantom sweating, gustatory sweating, Horner syndrome, and neuralgia. Compensatory sweating in other regions can occur in up to 90% of patients undergoing this procedure. The compensatory sweating is generally mild but has been reported to be severe in up to 40% of patients. Patients in this category generally prefer their premorbid condition over the compensatory hyperhidrosis. Recurrence rates following ETS have been reported in up to 2% of patients and immediate postsympathectomy failure rates are in the range of 0–2%. Failure rates have been attributed to a failure to ablate or resect the second thoracic ganglion; however, recent literature has also shown that preservation of this second thoracic ganglion may lead to a reduction in the incidence of compensatory sweating. Because compensatory sweating is usually irreversible and can be severely debilitating to patients, this necessitates explicit and detailed counseling of patients prior to undertaking this surgical procedure. Newer techniques include the use of clips instead of complete transsection of the nerve but reversal is not always possible as nerve destruction can be quick and compensatory disease may not be immediate. At present, the role for ETS appears to be in patients with palmar or axillary hyperhidrosis who have failed all other therapeutic modalities, including BTX.

BTX treatment

Multiple studies have validated the efficacy of BTX for the treatment of hyperhidrosis. Intradermal injections are clearly safe and well-tolerated and represent a viable alternative in the treatment of hyperhidrosis. BTX is produced by the anaerobic bacterium *Clostridium botulinum*. Seven different botulinum neurotoxins have been identified; however, BTX-A appears to be the most potent and is currently available as two commercial preparations (Botox®, Allergen Inc., Irvine, CA, USA; Dysport®, Ipsen, Berkshire, UK). One unit of Botox is estimated to be equal to 3–4 units of Dysport. The mechanism of action of BTX involves the inhibition of acetylcholine release at the neuromuscular junction and in cholinergic autonomic neurons. BTX injection results in a localized, prolonged, yet reversible, decrease in

cholinergic transmission. BTX-B (Myobloc) has also been used in a few studies for the treatment of hyperhidrosis. It seems to have a faster onset of action and greater diffusion. A higher incidence of local and systemic side effects have limited its use in the treatment of hyperhidrosis.

BTX for axillary hyperhidrosis

BTX for the treatment of axillary hyperhidrosis has been evaluated by two large randomized, controlled clinical trials in 465 patients. One trial in 145 patients with axillary hyperhidrosis unresponsive to topical therapy, defined as a rate of sweat production greater than 50 mg/min were randomized to BTX-A 200 units (Dysport) or placebo. After a 2-week period, the treatments were revealed and the axilla treated with placebo was injected with 100 units of BTX. Overall, there was an 81.4% decrease in sweat production with 200 units and a 76.5% decrease with 100 units; however, follow-up measurements of the rates of sweat production showed no advantage with the higher dosage. Sixty-three per cent of patients reported being completely satisfied, 29% reported being satisfied, and 8% reported being partially satisfied. Of note is the fact that 98% of patients stated they would recommend this treatment to others. BTX-A (Botox) was evaluated in another randomized, controlled study with 320 axillary hyperhidrosis patients. Patients were treated with either 50 units of BTX-A or placebo in each axilla. Treatment assessments were done at baseline and 16 weeks' post-treatment. Overall, the trial reported an 89% response rate at 1 week and a 93% response rate throughout the rest of the study period. During the post-treatment period dramatic and statistically significant improvements were noted in the treatment group with respect to various quality of life measures such as emotional status, ability to participate in daily and social activities, productivity at work, and number of clothing changes per day. Pain associated with these intradermal injections is reported to be minimal but a topical anesthetic can be used to further minimize the discomfort. Several smaller noncontrolled studies have also validated the above results in patients with axillary hyperhidrosis. BTX-A is a safe, well-tolerated, and highly efficacious treatment for axillary hyperhidrosis in patients who have failed to respond to topical therapy. The mean duration of effect is 6–7 months.

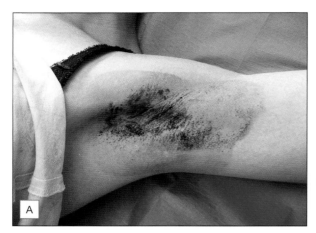
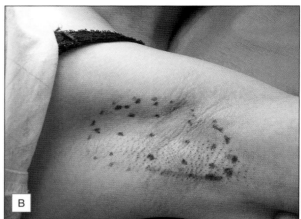

Fig. 9.3 (**A**) Starch iodine of axilla premarking. (**B**) Marking of affected area and sites of injection

Injection procedure

As noted above, specific studies on BTX-A for axillary hyperhidrosis have used different preparations (BOTOX or Dysport), different dosages, and different dilution techniques. BOTOX should be diluted with preserved normal saline (containing benzyl alcohol) in order to decrease the pain on injection. Different dilutions have been suggested for use in hyperhidrosis; however, a range of 2.5–5.0 cc is commonly used for every 100 units or vial of Botox. Dosages for injection range from 50 to 200 units/axilla. The usual starting dose is 50 units/axilla. It seems that the dose may have more to do with the distribution of drug in the given area of disease rather than the degree of disease severity. Larger surface areas of involvement may require more drug. A starch iodine test should be done to properly delineate the affected area. This will increase the accuracy of injection and results. As mentioned earlier, the area should be thoroughly dried and iodine solution (1–5%) should be evenly spread over the entire vault. Starch should then be sprinkled lightly over the area and the area of purple–black discoloration marked. This area can be further delineated with a surgical pen if needed. A digital picture can be helpful for future injections and monitoring efficacy.

After the area requiring treatment has been delineated (Fig. 9.3A), the drug is injected intradermally using a half-inch 30-gauge needle. This should be administered in a grid-like pattern in order to cover the entire area of involvement. Spacing should be approximately 1–2 cm apart (Fig. 9.3B). Some will mark injection sites to ensure the drug is distributed evenly throughout the treatment area. To minimize discomfort, topical anesthetics may be used ahead of time but may alter the effectiveness of the starch iodine test. It is also recommended to change the needle if it becomes dull. Side effects include rare bruising and minimal discomfort.

BTX for palmar hyperhidrosis

Two randomized, double-blind studies have evaluated the efficacy of BTX-A in palmar hyperhidrosis. A total of 30 patients were treated, with an overall response rate of greater than 90%. One study was with Dysport 120 mU diluted with 0.5 mL of 0.9% sterile saline and injected subcutaneously into one palm. Another bilateral paired second study used Botox 100 units diluted with 1.5 mL of 0.9% sterile saline, injected intradermally into each palm. The main side effects were pain at the site of injection and transient minor weakness of intrinsic hand muscles lasting 2–5 weeks with the Dysport but not with the Botox study. Other studies have reported a minor weakness of finger grip in two-thirds of patients. Patients have reported resolution of the reduced grip strength in days to weeks. Other noncontrolled trials have validated the high efficacy rate and safety of BTX-A in palmar hyperhidrosis. The duration of effect generally exceeded the length of the trials and is reported to be an average of 4–6 months.

Techniques and dosages of BTX-A differ among the studies for palmar hyperhidrosis as well. Intradermal injections spaced approximately 1–2 cm apart appear to give the best results (Fig. 9.4). It

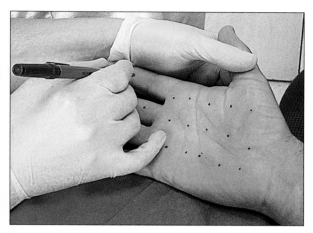

Fig. 9.4 Markings of injection sites for palmar injections

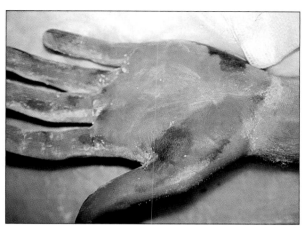

Fig. 9.5 Starch iodine of hand 2 weeks after treatment with BTX-A

seems to be more efficacious to treat palm size, adjusting for dose and number of injections based on surface area of involvement, rather than having a standard number of injection sites. A starch iodine test may not be required when injecting the palms when the entire surface area is involved. In the opinion of the authors, 100 units of Botox are enough for either palm but up to 200 units may be required for larger extremities. Spacing should be 2 cm apart and approximately 2 units of Botox are injected per site as required. Smaller syringes facilitate administration of the drug into this thick dermis. The use of a 50- or 100-unit insulin syringe with an ultrafine needle allows for easier injection and less spillage or reverse flow of the BTX out of the dermis. BTX-A injections for palmar hyperhidrosis represent a highly efficacious treatment alternative in patients who have failed to respond to topical therapies or iontophoresis (Fig. 9.5). The main limitation of this treatment method is the fact that most patients find the injections quite painful and therefore require regional nerve blocks. Side effects include bruising, mild discomfort and, rarely, temporary weakness of intrinsic hand muscles.

Regional anesthesia is achieved by a median, ulnar, and radial nerve block at the level of the wrist. The median nerve is located medial to the flexor carpi radialis tendon and just below the palmaris longus tendon at the level of the wrist crease. A skin wheal is raised at this site to block the palmar cutaneous branch of the median nerve. The needle is subsequently placed between the tendons. A total of 3–5 mL of local anesthetic (1% lidocaine) is injected approximately 0.5 cm below the surface. The ulnar nerve is located radial to the flexor carpi ulnaris. To block this nerve, the needle is inserted medial to the tendon, directing the needle towards the ulnar styloid. The superficial branch of the radial nerve can also be anesthetized by placing local anesthetic subcutaneously lateral to the radial artery as it extends towards the dorsum of the wrist or simply within the anatomic snuff box. It is very important that if any pain is felt in the distribution of the nerves when passing the needle into the wrist or upon injection of the anesthetic, it must be assumed that the needle has entered the nerve. The needle must be withdrawn and redirected to avoid neural damage. Patients should be warned that they cannot drive until the anesthesia has resolved.

The Bier block, which involves the insertion of a venous catheter into a distal vein, and application of a tourniquet followed by the injection of an anesthetic into the vein has been demonstrated to be superior to regional block anesthesia for plantar hyperhidrosis. This technique is reported to provide excellent pain control for palmar hyperhidrosis as well. This procedure usually requires the expertise of an anesthesiologist.

Recent reports of high intensity vibration in the areas of injection have significantly reduced injection pain. These devices held against the palms during injections are reasonably effective in minimizing pain.

BTX for plantar hyperhidrosis

There are currently no randomized, controlled trials evaluating BTX-A in plantar hyperhidrosis. Small case series and reports have demonstrated efficacy and improvement with dosages similar to those used in palmar studies, with a duration of effect between 4 and 6 months. Regional nerve block is generally required for anesthesia and involves the posterior tibial and sural nerves. A sural nerve block is achieved by injecting 3–5 mL of local anesthetic (1% lidocaine) subcutaneously between the lateral malleolus and the Achilles tendon. A posterior tibial nerve block uses a point located midway between the Achilles tendon and the medial malleolus. The needle is passed medially towards the tibia where approximately 5 mL of local anesthetic is injected. Following a nerve block, patients may have some instability when walking and cannot drive until the anesthesia has resolved. The authors have again used high-intensity vibration devices during the injection of BTX with acceptable pain control in some patients. A starch iodine test is usually recommended for the feet as the entire surface area may not be affected. The technique of injections is the same as for the palms. BTX represents a treatment alternative in patients with plantar hyperhidrosis who have failed topical therapy and iontophoresis. It is, however, often less successful than for axillary or palmar areas.

BTX for facial hyperhidrosis

Facial hyperhidrosis can involve the upper lip, nasolabial folds, and malar regions; however, the most commonly affected area is the forehead. Efficacy of BTX-A for facial hyperhidrosis is largely limited to case reports. Treatment with BTX has resulted in excellent results, with a duration of effect in the range of 5–6 months. The main site of injection is usually a band near the hairline. Frey's syndrome or facial gustatory sweating after parotid surgery or trauma is due to transection of the post-ganglionic sympathetic nerve fibers from the otic ganglion. Treatment with BTX-A has produced clinically significant results and improvements in associated facial flushing, lasting up to 15 months.

Treatment considerations with BTX

The main contraindications to BTX therapy include neuromuscular disorders such as myasthenia gravis, pregnancy and lactation, organic causes of hyperhidrosis, and medications that may interfere with neuromuscular transmission. Appropriate selection of patients and clinical presentations is essential to ensure a satisfactory treatment response and avoid unnecessary frustrations.

Summary

Hyperhidrosis is a common and extremely distressing condition, with a prevalence of 2.8% of the population. Approximately 50% of patients report feeling depressed. The fact that effective treatment, particularly BTX-A injections, can dramatically improve a patient's quality of life underscores the challenge for physicians to diagnose and manage this condition.

Further Reading

Furlan AD, Mailis A, Papagapiou M 2000 Are we paying a high price for surgical sympathectomy? A systematic literature review of late complications. Journal of Pain 1:245–257

Glogau RG 1998 Botulinum A neurotoxin for axillary hyperhidrosis. Dermatological Surgery 24(8):817–819

Hayton MJ, Stanley JK, Lowe NJ 2003 Local anaesthetic methods in the management of palmar hyperhidrosis: a review and description of treatment. British Journal of Dermatology 149:447–451

Heckmann M, Ceballos-Baumann AO, Plewig G 2001 Botulinum toxin A for axillary hyperhidrosis (excessive sweating). New England Journal of Medicine 344(7):488–493

Heckmann M, Teichmann B, Pause BM, Plewig G 2003 Amelioration of body odor after intracutaneous axillary injection of botulinium toxin A. Archives of Dermatology 139(1):57–59

Hornberger J, Grimes K, Naumann M, et al 2004 Recognition, diagnosis and treatment of primary focal hyperhidrosis. Journal of American Academy of Dermatology S1:274–286

Lowe NJ, Yamauchi PS, Lask GP, et al 2002 Efficacy and safety of botulinum toxin type A in the treatment of palmar hyperhidrosis: a double-blind, randomized, placebo-controlled study. Dermatological Surgery 28(9):822–827

Lowe PL, Cerdan-Sanz S, Lowe NJ 2004 Botulinum toxin type A in the treatment of bilateral primary axillary hyperhidrosis; efficacy and duration with repeated treatments. Dermatological Surgery, in press

Naumann M, Lowe NJ (on behalf of the BOTOX Hyperhidrosis Clinical Study Group) 2001 Botulinum toxin type A in treatment of bilateral primary axillary hyperhidrosis: randomised, parallel group, double-blind, placebo-controlled trial. British Medical Journal 323:1–4

Naumann M, Hamm H, Lowe NJ (on behalf of the BOTOX Hyperhidrosis Clinical Study Group) 2002 Effect of botulinum toxin type A on quality of life measures in patients with excessive axillary sweating: a randomised controlled trial. British Journal of Dermatology 147:1–9

Naumann M, Lowe NJ, Kumar CR, Hamm H (on behalf of the BOTOX Hyperhidrosis Clinical Study Group) 2003 Botulinum toxin type A is a safe and effective treatment for axillary hyperhidrosis over 16 months: a prospective study. Archives of Dermatology 139:731–736

Proebstle TM, Schneiders V, Knop J 2002 Gravimetrically controlled efficacy of sucorial curettage: a prospective study for treatment of axillary hyperhidrosis. Dermatological Surgery 28(11):1022–1026

Reinauer S, Neusser A, Schauf G, Hölzle E 1993 Iontophoresis with alternating current and direct current offset (AC/DC iontophoresis): a new approach for the treatment of hyperhidrosis. British Journal of Dermatology 129:166–169

Strutton DR, Kowalski JW, Glaser DA et al 2004 US prevalence of hyperhidrosis and impact on individuals with axillary hyperhidrosis: results from a national survey. Journal of American Academy of Dermatology S1:241–248

Zacherl J, Huber ER, Imhof M, et al 1998 Long-term results of 630 thoracoscopic sympathicotomies for primary hyperhidrosis: the Vienna experience. European Journal of Surgery 580(suppl): S43–46

10 Botulinum Toxin for Pain Relief and Treatment of Headache

Kevin C. Smith, Murad Alam

Introduction and Mechanisms of Action for Pain Relief

Since the 1985 report by Tsui et al that botulinum neurotoxin type-A (BTX-A) reduced the pain associated with torticollis, the list of painful conditions for which botulinum toxin (BTX) has been reported to be effective has been growing at a rapid rate (Box 10.1). Our understanding of the mechanisms of action of BTX-A for the management of pain has improved as a result of laboratory work as well as clinical experience

BTX-A blocks not only the release of acetylcholine from vesicles in nerve terminals, but also has been shown to inhibit the release from nerve endings of the pain-mediating neurotransmitter substance-P, which is known to play a role in some cases of postherpetic neuralgia. Administration of BTX-A may also reduce pain by blocking the presynaptic release of calcitonin gene-related peptide (CGRP), and through other mechanisms of action. Specifically, it has been suggested that these less understood effects may account for much of BTX-A treatment's antinociceptive benefits, such as blocking of peripheral sensitization and indirect reduction of central sensitization. Increasingly, it appears that complex BTX-A initiated central nervous system modifications may be crucial elements of the pain relief cascade.

Overview of Treatment Strategy

The remainder of this chapter will discuss the practical issues associated with the use of BTX-A for the management of three relatively common painful conditions: headache, painful scars, and postherpetic neuralgia; plus one uncommon condition, reflex sympathetic dystrophy. Also included is a discussion of the reported cases of BTX-associated headaches.

It is important to note that, in most cases, the formulation of BTX-A used for management of pain has been a specific commercial product available in the USA (Botox®, Allergan Corp., Irvine, CA, USA) which may not be directly comparable in dosage and action to other type A variants or other (e.g. type B) serotypes. The material referred to in this chapter was exclusively Botox®, and the doses are in units of Botox®.

Conditions where BTX-A or BTX-B treatment had led to pain relief
Anal fissure
Cervical dystonia
Cervicogenic headache
Chronic paroxysmal hemicrania
Chronic prostatic pain
Cluster headache
Dystonia-complex regional pain syndrome/reflex sympathetic dystrophy
Fibromyalgia
Headache
Interstitial cystitis
Intractable spasmodic torticollis
Low back pain
Migraine headache
Muscle tension headache
Myofascial pain
Pericranial pain syndromes
Peripheral neuropathy
Phantom pain following amputation
Postherpetic neuralgia
Pyriformis syndrome
Relapsing-remitting multiple sclerosis
Severe tingling caused by herniation of cervical vertebrae
Temporomandibular disorders
Trigeminal neuralgia
Whiplash

Box 10.1 Conditions where BTX-A or BTX-B treatment had led to pain relief

Treatment of Muscle Tension, Migraine, and Other Types of Headache

The three most common forms of headache—tension headache, migraine headache, and cluster headache—have each been reported by at least some authors to respond well to BTX-A. In clinical practice, it is common to encounter patients whose headaches overlap somewhat between these three classic types of headache.

Patients who should be considered for BTX-A therapy of headaches include those who demonstrate a lack of improvement from preventive (prophylactic) pharmacotherapy; those who experience severe and intolerable adverse events from preventive medications; those who refuse daily medications; and those who have contraindications to acute migraine therapy. In addition, BTX-A therapy may simply be preferable and less expensive or have fewer side-effects than other treatments and so be considered for first-line therapy. However, an accurate diagnosis must be made, ideally by someone skilled in the differential diagnosis of headache.

Hu et al have shown that the economic burden of migraine predominantly falls on patients and their employers in the form of bedridden days and lost productivity. Hence, it is useful clinically, for communication with other physicians and third party payers, to objectively quantify patients' pretreatment condition and degree of response to therapy. Objective measures which may facilitate documentation of headache treatments include:

- Likert pain scale and global assessment (Fig. 10.1)
- physician's global assessment (Fig. 10.2)
- number of doses of headache or pain medication taken in the past 30 days (diary)
- MIDAS score (measures headache effect on employment and activities of daily living) (see http://www.migraine-disability.net/About_Midas/default.asp)
- HIT-6 index (measures headache effect on employment and activities of daily living) (see http://www.headachetest.com/HIT6/PDFS/English.pdf)

It is also useful to collect the baseline history in a systematic manner (Fig. 10.3) and to record the location and dose of the injections in a standardized manner (Fig. 10.4).

While a minority of patients will experience very dramatic relief of their headaches within hours or days, it is more typical for patients to improve in a stepwise manner, with as many as 80% of patients in some series achieving a high level of relief after four to five treatments. Because treatment with BTX-A will usually control but not cure headaches, and because improvement is usually incremental, it is important to determine whether or not the patient or third party payer can afford BTX-A treatments before embarking on a course of therapy.

While some dermatologists are highly skilled in the administration of BTX-A, investigation of the pathophysiology of headaches and the management of other headache medication should usually be left to the patient's primary physician or neurologist. This division of labor is reasonable, given dermatologists' technical expertise in the administration of BTX-A but their limited training regarding the investigation and differential diagnosis of headache.

The dosage of BTX-A, the locations of the injections, and the frequency of treatment are all tailored to the specific patient while remaining within certain commonly accepted parameters. In general, the patient is encouraged to continue with the current program of medications for migraine (for example acetaminophen, nonsteroidal anti-inflammatories, and triptans) until it becomes possible to gradually reduce those medications as the effects of BTX-A treatment emerge. Patients are also encouraged to identify and, as much as possible, avoid factors that trigger their headaches (for example smoking, noise or certain foods).

Often the most efficient way to administer BTX-A is to have the patient identify the areas from which pain originates and to which it radiates. This can be accomplished by having the patient make a fingernail mark at the point of maximal discomfort. (Without this instruction, patients may point with several fingers to the general area of discomfort.) Each of the areas identified by the patient are then injected, usually with aliquots of between 4 and 12 units of BTX-A/injection site, with injections spaced 1.5–3 cm apart. For example, treatment of the right parietal area would typically require three to four injections, with a total dose between 12 and 48 units of BTX-A. This 'follow the pain' approach can sometimes produce satisfactory results using relatively small quantities of BTX-A. In cases where the cost of BTX-A is not an obstacle, injection placement in the configurations illustrated in Figures 10.5–10.7 may be more efficacious than a pure 'follow the pain' approach, and this can be further enhanced by injecting extra BTX-A into specific problem areas.

Last name   First name   Chart #   Date

Patient's rating scale:

Please circle the number which best describes the amount of pain you are having today in the involved area:

When you are not touching the area

NO pain   0   1   2   3   4   5   6   7   8   9   10   WORST possible pain

When the area is touched or rubbed

NO pain   0   1   2   3   4   5   6   7   8   9   10   WORST possible pain

---

Please circle the number which best describes whether your PAIN in the involved area is BETTER or WORSE compared with how it was at your last visit:

BETTER   5   4   3   2   1   0   1   2   3   4   5   WORSE

Please circle the number which best describes your OVERALL impression of how you are doing compared with the previous visit

BETTER   5   4   3   2   1   0   1   2   3   4   5   WORSE

Fig. 10.1 Patient's Likert scales for pain and overall status. These scales can be repeated at every visit

Occasionally, patients will identify areas of involvement on the scalp where there are few muscle fibers available for injection. These areas usually respond as well as more muscular areas to injections of BTX-A, supporting the suggestion that the benefits of BTX-A treatment in headache derive at least in part from mechanisms other than direct muscle relaxation.

In areas that are cosmetically important (for example, the face and forehead) it is necessary to inject in a symmetrical manner so that muscle relaxation on both sides of the face and forehead will be equal, and facial symmetry will be preserved. Another reason to maintain symmetry (even in noncosmetic areas like the parietal and nuchal muscles) is to reduce the chance that discomfort will be unmasked on the contralateral side after the most painful primary areas of concern have been treated. Anecdotally, it has been noted that in noncosmetic areas it is sometimes adequate to treat the asymptomatic side with only 50% of the dose used on the symptomatic

side. For example, if a patient notes that migraines usually start in the left parietal area, a sufficient treatment might consist of four doses of 8 units of BTX-A to the left parietalis muscle and four doses of 4 units of BTX-A into the right parietalis muscle.

When tension headache is a major component of the problem, a patient may identify discomfort in either one or both of the masseter muscles. In such cases, both masseters are injected with three to five 8- to 12-unit doses of Botox, using a 30 gauge, 1 inch (2.5-cm) needle. As with other injections for pain or headache, it is recommended that the patient participate by identifying the precise loci of discomfort. When the masseters are injected, it may be beneficial to also inject the temporo-parietal muscles with three or four 4- to 12-unit doses on each side. If there is masseter involvement, palpation of the internal pterygoid muscles (in the posterior part of the mouth, posterior to the upper and lower molars) is indicated. Should the pterygoids be tender,

---

Last name   First name   Chart #   Date

Physician's rating scale:

Please circle the number which best describes the amount of pain the patient appears to be having today in the involved area:

When the area is not touched

    NO pain   0   1   2   3   4   5   6   7   8   9   10   WORST possible pain

When the area is touched or rubbed

    NO pain   0   1   2   3   4   5   6   7   8   9   10   WORST possible pain

---

Please circle the number which best describes whether the patient's pain in the involved area appears to be BETTER or WORSE compared with how it was at the patient's last visit:

    BETTER   5   4   3   2   1   0   1   2   3   4   5   WORSE

Please circle the number which best describes your overall impression of how this patient is doing compared with the previous visit

    BETTER   5   4   3   2   1   0   1   2   3   4   5   WORSE

Fig. 10.2 Physician's Likert scales for pain and overall status. These scales can be repeated at every visit

headache and/or masseter discomfort can be improved by injecting the internal pterygoids with 5–10 units of BTX-A on each side.

Where there is a cervicogenic component to the headaches, the patient will often identify areas of involvement in the posterior neck and upper back. These are typically injected with 5–10 units every 1.5–3 cm on the affected side, with about half that dose delivered to the contralateral, clinically asymptomatic side. Until the patient's response to therapy has been determined, to reduce the risk of weakness the total dose in the nuchal muscles should be limited to no more than 60 units per session via a 30 gauge, 1 inch needle.

For pain in or behind the eyes, injection is appropriate into the muscles around the eyes, including the procerus, depressor supercilii, corrugators, lateral orbicularis occuli, and nasalis. Injection of the inferior orbicularis occuli (inferior to the margin of the lower eyelid) has not been helpful.

Individuals treated for headache may be invited to return for follow-up 2–3 weeks after their first treatment for assessment of the results. Additional BTX-A treatments are typically given at 6- to 10-week intervals, depending on the needs of the patient. Patients not infrequently return for more BTX-A injections while the injected muscles are still very flaccid from the previous treatment. This lends further credence to the theory that BTX-A injections prevent pain by mechanisms other than, or in addition to, muscle relaxation. There is less concern now than in the past about the possibility of antibodies developing against BTX-A if patients are treated frequently (perhaps more often than every 8 weeks) and/or at high doses (for example, over 100 units per treatment). Jankovic et al found that blocking antibodies were detected in four of 42 (9.5%) cervical dystonia patients treated only with the original formulation of Botox® but in none of the 119 patients ($p < 0.004$) treated exclusively

---

Botox Therapeutic™ Headache Screening

Last name _____   First name _____   Chart # _____   Date _____

1. Have you ever had a diagnosis made regarding your headaches, for example 'migraine' or 'muscle tension headache'?

2. How **long** have you had your headaches?

   How **often** do you have headaches?

3. Are you sensitive to loud noises when you have a headache?   Yes ____   No ____

   Are you sensitive to bright lights when you have a headache?   Yes ____   No ____

   Do you sometimes have nausea when you have a headache?   Yes ____   No ____

   Do you sometimes have vomiting when you have a headache?   Yes ____   No ____

4. Do you know of anything that brings your headaches on, for example changes in the weather, menses, certain foods etc.?

5. Has anyone in your family had headaches like yours?

6. What area is most painful when you have a headache?

    Second most painful?

7. Which medications or other treatments have you tried for your headaches?

8. What treatments have you been using in the past month?

   Please list the number of doses of each medicine taken in the past 30 days:

9. Have you seen any specialists (for example, a neurologist) for your headaches?

   If yes, who?

10. Have you had any tests (for example, a CT or MRI scan of the head)?

Fig. 10.3 BTX-A headache screening questionnaire. This questionnaire provides helpful baseline information regarding a headache patient who is considering a trial of treatment with BTX

with the current formulation of Botox®, which has been on the market since late 1997.

While some patients at least initially may require or desire treatment every 4–8 weeks, there are other fortunate patients who receive treatments at 6- to 8-month intervals. Some of these people have headaches mainly triggered by changes in the weather, and so require treatment mainly in the spring and possibly again in the autumn.

Patients with a pre-existing headache history will occasionally have an exacerbation of headaches after BTX-A treatment. This may occur as a result of irritation from injections or, more often, the natural temporal fluctuations in the clinical course of the

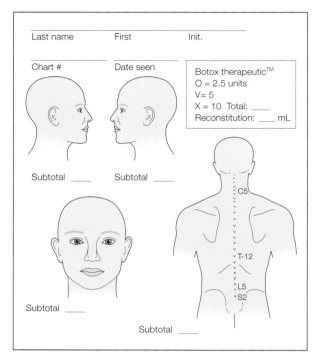

Fig. 10.4 BTX-A headache treatment record. This treatment record facilitates accurate recording of the doses and locations of BTX injections for headache and for pain in the mid and lower back

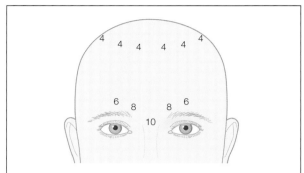

Fig. 10.5 Typical doses of BTX-A for headache involving the forehead and glabellar complex

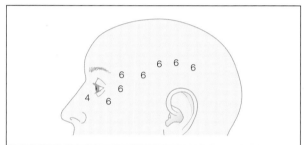

Fig. 10.6 Typical doses of BTX-A for headaches involving the temporoparietal area and nasalis

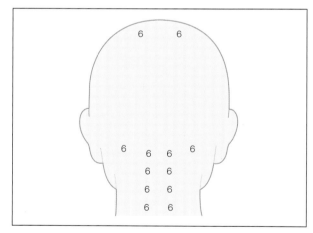

Fig. 10.7 Typical doses of BTX-A for headaches involving the occipitalis and nuchal areas

underlying disease. Some reports suggest that patients with coexisting chronic fatigue syndrome and/or fibromyalgia may have a higher incidence of headache after injection of BTX-A injection into the face, forehead, neck or scalp than do members of the general population. Headache induction may also be technique dependent and related to needle trauma. In at least a small series, diminished headache induction has followed replacing a 0.8 cm Becton-Dickinson BD-II 30 gauge diabetic needle/syringe combination with the somewhat finer 1.3 cm SteriJect 31 gauge needle mounted on a 1 mL Henke Dose Saver syringe (both available from www.air-tite.com in Virginia Beach, VA, USA). In addition to potentially reducing discomfort, the extra length of 31 gauge SteriJect needles facilitates injection of the deeper muscles of the temporoparietal and nuchal areas with reduced bleeding and bruising.

Possible Induction of Headaches

BTX-A injections have been used not only to treat headache but have also on rare occasions been associated with the development of headache. The well-known but quite uncommon effect of mild, transient headache can manifest following injection of BTX-A for dynamic creases of the upper face. Typically, the headache lasts a few days to a week and remits spontaneously.

The first report of long-lasting headache after injection was published in 2001. In a case series of several hundred consecutive patients treated for cosmetic improvement of the forehead, glabella, and crow's feet, the authors noted an approximately 1% incidence of persistent headache lasting up to several months. Interestingly, the said headaches occurred exclusively in patients without any pre-existing history of tension or migraine headaches.

Since the initial report of long-lasting BTX-related headaches, there have been few additional reports of similar headaches. Further, the authors of the first report (personal communication) are also aware of only a small number of unpublished cases. The estimated incidence of long-lasting headaches is thus likely much lower than the original estimate of 1%, and given the ubiquity of BTX-A treatments for wrinkles, long-lasting headaches are probably best described as rare rather than merely uncommon. When protracted headaches do occur, their induction may be technique-dependent, related to the process of needle insertion rather than a pharmacologic effect of BTX-A; it has been shown that needling of the forehead independent of injection of any fluid can elicit headache.

At present, the informed consent process for BTX-A injection for cosmetic effect need not include discussion of persistent headaches. The rarity of this association, coupled with its essentially benign and fully remitting course, suggests that it is of primarily academic interest.

Treatment of Postherpetic Neuralgia

In several series, BTX-A has been successfully used to treat patients with chronic, intractable postherpetic neuralgia (PHN) in the trigeminal distribution. As is the case when treating headaches, treatment may be directed more precisely using objective measures to quantify the response to therapy. For instance, at multiple time points, the patient may complete the Likert Scale for Pain and a global assessment measure (Fig. 10.1) and the physician may complete a physician version of the Likert Scale as well as a global assessment (Fig. 10.2). These subjective measures may be correlated with estimates of both the number of doses of pain medication taken in the week prior to the visit. PHN patients may continue with their current pain medications concurrently with BTX-A treatment and only gradually reduce those medications once they begin to

experience benefits from BTX-A treatment. In at least one case a patient with chronic, severe PHN on the trunk responded almost completely to BTX-A injections, stopped her pain medications abruptly, and developed symptoms of narcotic withdrawal (Dr M. Sapijaszko, personal communication, St Anton, Austria, February 2004).

Prior to injections for PHN, the patient identifies the area or areas of involvement, the boundaries of which may then be marked with washable pink fluorescent marker and photographed (Fig. 10.8). Injections of BTX-A may be placed intradermally or subdermally in quantities of 2.5–5 units/injection, and spacing of 2–3 cm apart; the total dose is typically approximately 1–2 units/cm². Intradermal and subdermal injections seem to be equally effective, but when treating the face and forehead the BTX-A is usually injected intradermally, to minimize unwanted muscle relaxation, which may still occur to some extent.

To reduce injection discomfort further, it may be decided to reconstitute BTX-A for injection into PHN using normal saline with benzyl alcohol preservative (which has local anesthetic properties). There is no consensus as to the optimal reconstitution volume for this indication, but there is some agreement regarding the overall doses in terms of units delivered. Because there is commonly hyperalgesia in the involved area, use of fine 31 gauge SteriJect needles may reduce discomfort. While it is not common practice to pretreat patients with topical anesthetics, this may be considered in cases of potentially intolerable injection discomfort.

The antinociceptive effect of BTX-A seems to peak at about 3 weeks, so patients may return for reassessment and possible retreatment every 3–4 weeks. The usual number of treatments required to induce long-term remission of PHN ranges from 1 to 4.

Serial photography of ink-marked PHN lesions tends to reveal a reduction in the surface area of involvement as the patient responds to BTX-A injections. A paradoxical increase in the visual-analog pain score in the residual area(s) of involvement may occur as the total area of involvement shrinks and as the patient's and physician's global assessment improves. This phenomenon is not understood, but it has been speculated that the mildest areas of discomfort resolve first in response to BTX-A treatment, and when these mild areas are no longer 'averaged' with the more severe areas by the patient, the visual-analog pain score in the residual areas

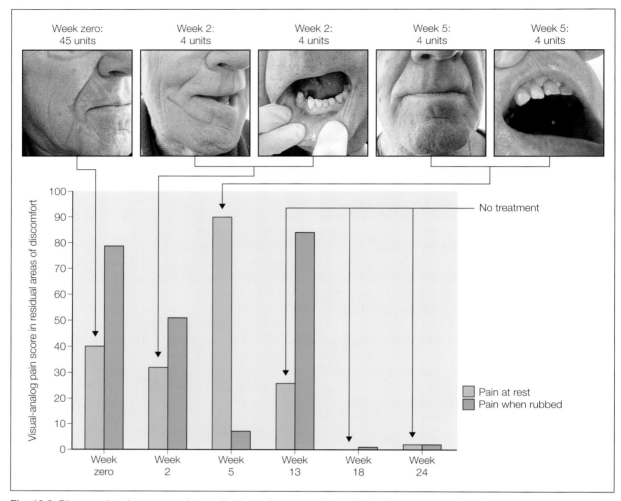

Fig. 10.8 Diagram showing progressive decline in surface area affected by PHN, and eventual elimination of pain after transient increase in visual-analog pain scores in residual areas of PHN

rises. Irritation from mild areas of involvement may also activate a 'gating' mechanism at the level of the spinal cord that limits the severity of the pain signals crossing the midline and ascending along a final common pathway to the sensorium.

When the PHN patient is rendered pain-free, there is frequently a long-term drug-free remission of pain. The reasons for this are also poorly understood. It may be that the same plasticity of the nervous system which is postulated to facilitate the development of chronic pain may also facilitate the resolution of chronic pain after treatment with BTX-A (Figs 10.9 and 10.10).

Treatment of Painful Scars

BTX-A has been reported in case series to be useful for treating pain associated with keloids, hypertrophic scars, and uncomplicated scars. The treatment of painful scars with BTX-A has evolved more recently than other indications, such as headaches and PHN. Significantly, the general therapeutic approach is similar, with serial ratings of the degree of discomfort, followed by marking of the area, photography, and finally injection (Fig. 10.11). In the case of a thick scar (for example, a keloid on the central chest after thoracotomy), the patient may offer advice about whether the pain is deep or superficial and the injection can be adjusted to take this into account.

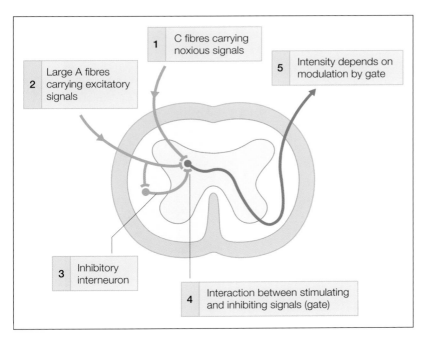

Fig. 10.9 Gate theory of pain control: plasticity of the nervous system

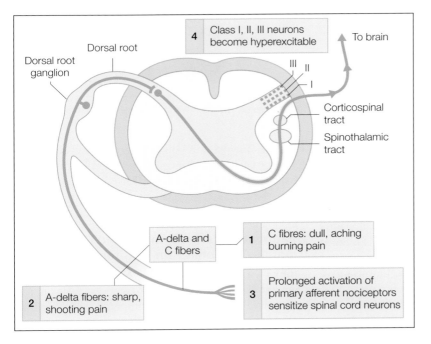

Fig. 10.10 Ascending pain pathways

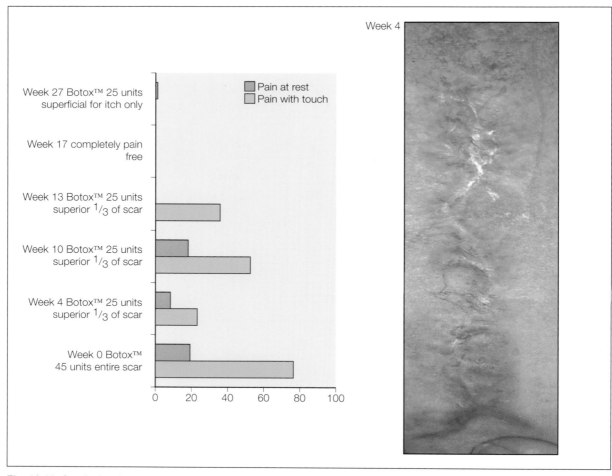

Fig. 10.11 Graph showing visual-analog pain scores in response to a course of treatment with BTX-A for painful sternal keloid

To minimize injection discomfort into raised, dense scars, a small injection volume is preferred, and a reconstitution of 1 mL/100 units BTX-A is preferred. If the scar is quite sensitive, injection discomfort can be reduced or eliminated by infiltrating the tissue around and under the scar with 1% or 2% lidocaine before BTX-A is injected into the scar. The amount of BTX-A administered in each treatment may range from 10 to 50 units/cm³ of scar tissue. Duration of remission, follow-up, and treatment intervals are as with treatment of PHN.

Some patients have noted no clinically significant improvement in the appearance (assessed by serial photography) of scars injected with BTX-A, but at least one hypertrophic scar on the breast seemed much softer 6 months after two injections. Because some of the peptides implicated in the mechanism of action of BTX-A may interact with some of the cytokines involved in collagen remodeling and collagen deposition, it is conceivable, albeit highly speculative, that treatment with BTX-A injections could affect the physical properties of some scars, perhaps with repeated treatments or after longer follow-up.

Treatment of Reflex Sympathetic Dystrophy (Complex Regional Pain Syndrome)

Reflex sympathetic dystrophy is characterized by constant burning pain and hyperesthesia in an extremity. Pain is often accompanied by swelling, sweating, vasomotor instability and, sometimes, trophic changes. There is often a history of injury or other trauma, and muscle spasms, myoclonus or focal dystonia may occur. Diffuse pain, loss of function, and autonomic dysfunction are three main criteria suggested for diagnosis. Successful use of BTX-A for relief of this condition has been reported.

One of the authors (KCS) has treated a 41-year-old woman with refractory reflex sympathetic dystrophy affecting the right arm after a motor vehicle accident 8 years' previously. The patient characterized her pain as coming predominantly from bone, and deep injections close to bone using a 30 gauge 1 inch needle were of particular benefit. Subcutaneous and intramuscular injections of BTX-A (a total of 120–400 units/session, about once a month) into the areas of discomfort in the right hand and arm gave substantial pain relief (for which the patient is very grateful) and have also normalized skin color and temperature in the right hand and forearm. However, 1 year of treatments have yet to produce any improvement in her ability to use the right hand. This is consistent with the observations of Cordivari et al, who noted that four out of four of their patients with dystonia-complex regional pain syndrome affecting the hand experienced pain relief after treatment with BTX-A (Dysport, Ipsan Inc., Berkshire, UK) but only one of the four had functional improvement.

Conclusions

In summary, there are a growing number of applications for BTX-A in the treatment of noncosmetic pain syndromes. Headache, one of the best studied such application, is mitigated by precisely targeting the muscle groups and foci of discomfort. Best results are usually obtained by choosing injection points in consultation with the individual being treated, and custom tailoring the injection locations and treatment schedule to the needs of that individual. After several treatment sessions there is usually marked and long-lasting control for migraine and tension headache sufferers, and sometimes those with more exotic headache syndromes.

A variety of other pain syndromes are now routinely treated with BTX-A injections. Notably, postherpetic neuralgia, painful scars, and reflex sympathetic dystrophy have been shown to improve or enter prolonged remission with treatment. Most of the evidence is in the form of case reports, but these are becoming sufficiently frequent that nonheadache pain syndromes are now a recognized off-label indication for BTX-A. At lest one clinical trial of BTX-A for postherpetic neuralgia is underway, as of December 2004.

It appears that the efficacy of BTX-A in pain disorders may derive from a combination of its known peripheral mechanism of action (blocking the release of substance-P and perhaps other neurotransmitters from neuronal vesicles) and perhaps also distinct central nervous system mechanisms. As the mechanisms of action of BTX for the relief and prevention of pain are elucidated, pain treatment protocols using BTX and other related neuromodulators will be refined and made more effective and efficient.

Further Reading

Alam M, Arndt KA, Dover JS 2002 Severe, intractable headache following injection with botulinum A exotoxin: report of five cases. Journal of the American Academy of Dermatology 46:62–65

Aoki KR, Aoki RK 2003 Evidence for antinociceptive activity of botulinum toxin type A in pain management. Headache 43(Suppl 1):S9–S15

Arezzo JC 2002 Possible mechanisms for the effects of botulinum toxin on pain. Clinical Journal of Pain 18(6 Suppl):S125–132

Argoff CE 2002 A focused review on the use of botulinum toxins for neuropathic pain. Clinical Journal of Pain 18(6 Suppl):S177–181

Bernstein JE, Bickers DR, Dahl MV, et al 1987 Treatment of chronic postherpetic neuralgia with topical capsaicin. A preliminary study. Journal of the American Academy of Dermatology 17(1):93–96

Brin MF, Binder W, Blitzer A, et al 2002 Botulinum toxin type A BOTOX® for pain and headache. In: Brin MF, Hallett M, Jankovic J (eds) Scientific and therapeutic aspects of botulinum toxin. Lippincott Williams and Wilkins, Philadelphia, pp. 233–250

Cordivari C, Misra VP, Catania S, et al 2001 Treatment of dystonic clenched fist with botulinum toxin. Movement Disorders 16(5):907–913

Crowe R, Parkhouse N, McGrouther D 1994 Neuropeptide-containing nerves in painful hypertrophic human scar tissue. British Journal of Dermatology 130(4):444–452

Hu XH, Markson LE, Lipton RB, et al 1999 Burden of migraine in the United States: disability and economic costs. Archives of Internal Medicine 159(8):813–818

Jankovic J, Vuong KD, Ahsan J 2003 Comparison of efficacy and immunogenicity of original versus current botulinum toxin in cervical dystonia. Neurology 60(7):1186–1188

Melzack R, Wall PD 1965 Pain mechanisms: a new theory. Science 150(699):971–979

Purkiss J, Welch M, Doward S, et al 2000 Capsaicin-stimulated release of substance P from cultured dorsal root ganglion neurons: involvement of two distinct mechanisms. Biochemical Pharmacology 59(11):1403–1406

Rumsfield JA, West DP 1991 Topical capsaicin in dermatologic and peripheral pain disorders. DICP 25(4):381–387

Saenz A, Avellanet M, Garreta R 2003 Use of botulinum toxin type A on orthopedics: a case report. Archives of Physical Medicine in Rehabilitation 84(7):1085–1086

Sala C, Andreose JS, Fumagalli G, et al 1995 Calcitonin gene-related peptide: possible role in formation and maintenance of neuromuscular junctions. Journal of Neuroscience 15(1 Pt 2):520–528

Tarabal O, Caldero J, Ribera J, et al 1996 Regulation of motoneuronal calcitonin gene-related peptide (CGRP) during axonal growth and neuromuscular synaptic plasticity induced by botulinum toxin in rats. European Journal of Neuroscience 8(4):829–836

Tsui JK, Eisen A, Mak E, et al 1985 A pilot study on the use of botulinum toxin in spasmodic torticollis. Canadian Journal of Neurological Science 12(4):314–316

Welch MJ, Purkiss JR, Foster KA 2000 Sensitivity of embryonic rat dorsal root ganglia neurons to Clostridium botulinum neurotoxins. Toxicon 38(2):245–258

Winner P 2003 Botulinum toxins in the treatment of migraine and tension-type headaches. Physical Medicine in Rehabilitation Clinics in North America 14(4):885–899

11

Treatment of Facial Asymmetry with Botulinum Toxin

J. Charles Finn, Sue Ellen Cox

Introduction

Facial symmetry is a key determinate in facial attractiveness. Preference for symmetrical faces appears to be 'hard wired' into the brain as even neonates exhibit preference for symmetrical faces. The preference for symmetry permeates throughout cultures and may have evolved as a mechanism for the selection of the ideal mate. As clinicians have developed years of experience utilizing botulinum toxin type A (BTX-A), the therapy has evolved from a treatment for wrinkles to a technique for facial reshaping. By understanding the agonist/antagonist relationship of the various facial muscles, the experienced injector can reliably reposition and reshape facial structures in carefully selected patients, restoring some degree of facial symmetry.

The problem being treated

There may be many causes for facial asymmetry. Underlying bone development is responsible for the majority of asymmetries. Typically, one side of the face is longer, creating a subtle curve to the face. There may also be differences in facial soft tissue volume, the most dramatic being hemifacial atrophy. Asymmetries from volume differences are best treated with craniofacial surgery, implants, or injectable soft tissue fillers. Asymmetries also develop from side-to-side differences in muscle function. Modern image analysis software is very useful in demonstrating subtle facial differences to patients. Experienced surgeons make a point of demonstrating these asymmetries to patients prior to surgical procedures, as meticulous patients invariably notice them following surgery. The same holds true for the cosmetic candidate for BTX-A therapy. The patient and physician should undergo a critical analysis of the patient's features prior to treatment. This dialog helps solidify treatment goals and possibilities while strengthening the patient–physician relationship.

Differences in muscle function stem from a variety of causes. Many develop due to malfunction or injury of the facial nerve, resulting in hypo-function or hyperfunction of the innervated muscle. Other muscle asymmetries may be functional in nature, e.g. the frontalis may be hyperfunctional to elevate a ptotic eyelid and improve visual field (Figs 11.1 & 11.2). Still other muscular asymmetries are merely habitual or idiopathic in nature (Fig. 11.3).

Facial nerve malfunctions emanate from multiple etiologies. Causes may be congenital, traumatic, infectious, neoplastic, neurological, or idiopathic. However, most facial nerve injuries are traumatic or due to Bell's palsy. Traumatic facial nerve injuries can be from blunt or sharp injury, and are often iatrogenic from otologic or oncologic surgery. Bell's palsy, or idiopathic facial nerve paralysis, is a diagnosis of exclusion. Bell's palsy affects an estimated 15–40 per 100 000 people per year. The majority of patients recover completely, but approximately 10% may have significant residual abnormality.

Nerve injuries may be partial or complete. Mild compression to the nerve causes decreased flow of axoplasm, leading to neuropraxia. This is a temporary functional deficit which will resolve within days to a few weeks after nerve compression is relieved. More severe compression injuries cause destruction and degeneration of the distal axon while the myelin sheath is preserved. This allows regeneration of the neural tubules through the original pathway. Recovery of this type of compression injury may take several months as the axon regenerates through the undamaged myelin sheath at a rate of 0.3 mm per day. Still, full functional recovery is likely.

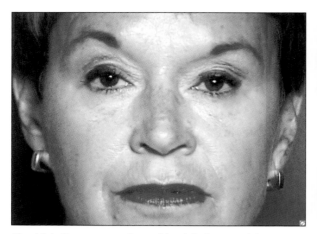

Fig. 11.1 Brow asymmetry and frontalis hyperactivity secondary to eyelid ptosis. This is a functional muscular hyperactivity

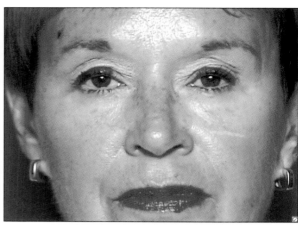

Fig. 11.2 After frontalis treatment, symmetry is restored, but subjective visual field is decreased. This patient depended on frontalis hyperactivity to aid her visual field and should not have been treated

With more severe compression or transection injury, not only do the distal axons degenerate, but the supporting neural tubules are disrupted as well. When the injured axon regenerates, it follows any available neural tubule with frequent misdirection. With these more severe injuries, recovery takes longer and is usually incomplete. Some of the reinnervated muscles receive weak neural input, some receive misguided input and some receive no input at all. Some muscles actually become hyperfunctional with excess resting tone or inappropriate contraction from misdirected axonal regeneration. Some muscles may remain hypotonic. With injury to the main trunk of the facial nerve, reinnervation will not be selective, resulting in some degree of synkinesis. Synkinesis results when facial muscles contract as a unit rather than individually. For example, the orbicularis oculi muscle will contract with mouth movements or the corner of the mouth will pull when squinting. Spasms and twitching are also common following nerve regeneration. If resting muscle tone varies from side-to-side, facial asymmetry will result. BTX-A therapy is helpful in treating many types of muscular facial asymmetries.

When a patient suffers a facial nerve injury from surgery or trauma, the ultimate degree of facial nerve injury is not always obvious with acute injury. Partial function implies nerve continuity and is a good prognostic sign. Full paralysis may be due to complete transection or only neuropraxia, with prompt resolution in a few weeks. If surgical exploration is

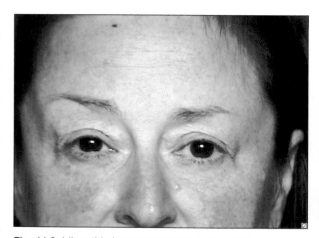

Fig. 11.3 Idiopathic brow asymmetry that would be a good candidate for BTX-A therapy

not indicated, facial symmetry may be temporarily enhanced by using BTX-A on the noninjured side. This is especially useful in injuries to the frontal or marginal branches, usually iatrogenic. In effect, one buys time for the injured branch to heal and recover.

With chronic injuries, the clinician may be presented with a mixture of hyperfunction, synkinesis, and hypofunction. Resting tone of muscles should be assessed first for asymmetry. In the brow region, a hypofunctional brow will show relative ptosis. Orbicularis oculi tone is very important for eye shape and lid position. A completely atonic lid may have incomplete closure and exposure keratitis. An orbicularis oculi muscle which is hypertonic with synkinesis will show a smaller ocular aperture. Resting mouth position should be assessed.

Patient selection and expected benefits

Careful patient selection is key for optimal results. BTX-A will certainly not improve a flaccid paralysis. However, if an isolated muscle is paretic, BTX-A treatment to the contralateral, normal muscle may improve symmetry and decrease the visual appearance of the paralysis. The frontal branch of the facial nerve is an excellent application of this technique. To some extent, paresis of the marginal branch of the facial nerve can respond to a similar treatment. In these cases, BTX-A is used to decrease tone on the normal side to improve asymmetry.

BTX-A treatment is also effective in treating hyperfunctional muscles. If a muscle is primarily hyperfunctional, i.e. hemifacial spasm or blepharospasm, large doses of BTX-A are necessary for effective treatment. If a muscle is hyperfunctional due to aberrant regeneration of an injured facial nerve, the muscle tends to be very sensitive to chemodenervation. Whether treating a normal muscle or a hyperfunctional muscle, treatment of facial asymmetry is a subtle art and patients need to be aware of the need for frequent touch-ups and retreatment. Individual patients respond in a variety of ways and careful documentation of injection site and dosage is key for reliable treatment.

Chemodenervation plays one role in a full program of facial nerve rehabilitation. Considerable improvement of the preinjury state may be obtainable; however, complete restoration is not possible. Chronically asymmetric patients are typically very satisfied with subtle improvements, while facial nerve injury patients may be understandably distressed about their condition and may have unreasonable expectations of treatment results. The treating physician should candidly discuss the examination findings with the patient to open a dialogue discussing the goals and limitations of treatment. It is imperative to discuss carefully the risks and benefits of the treatment and the anticipated outcome in order effectively to manage the patient's expectations. Thorough discussion with the patient should include the goals of treatment, whether it is improved symmetry at rest or improved symmetry with expression. Risks of treatment, including worsening of asymmetry, should be carefully considered. Patients should understand the temporary nature of BTX treatment as well as the fact that treatment should have no effect on the underlying disease. Dosages should be carefully titrated, often requiring multiple follow-up visits for touch-ups.

Treatment Techniques

Detailed understanding of facial muscle anatomy is paramount to successful treatment. The clinician should have exact understanding of each muscle's innervation and mimetic effect. Each muscle has an exact origin and insertion which leads to the movement of the overlying structures. Some patients will have pre-existing asymmetries to the facial bony or soft tissue anatomy, which may obfuscate abnormalities of the nerve, and should be noted. Careful, consistent photography is invaluable for objective documentation of the asymmetries.

Before considering treatment, the facial nerve should be methodically evaluated to understand the abnormality and the patterns of regeneration. First, resting tone should be assessed. Care should be taken to look at the face as a whole to assess for gross asymmetries as well as resting tone of each muscle group. Ocular aperture size, position of the mouth, brow and other features can offer clues to underlying muscle imbalance. Involuntary twitches or spasms should be noted. Following assessment of resting muscle tone, each muscle group should be examined at full forced contraction. This will often exaggerate the resting asymmetry of the paretic face. Any synkinesis should be noted as each group is evaluated as an isolated contraction. Surprisingly, many normal patients may have difficulty isolating specific muscle group contractions. While performing this examination, the practitioners should be considering the pattern of injury to various facial nerve branches. Following facial nerve injury, muscles may present with aberrant innervation. For example, in a patient with synkinesis, squinting will cause the corner of the mouth to be pulled to the affected side. Conversely, a forced smile will cause an involuntary squinting of the ipsilateral eye.

Last, and most important, is close observation of the face during animated conversation. Patients should be assessed in casual speech with natural social interaction. Patients are usually very aware of abnormalities that they can see in a mirror, but will not be aware of the dramatic asymmetries present

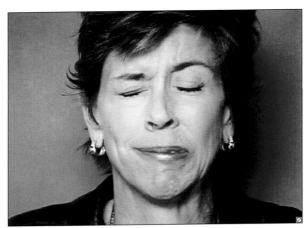

Fig. 11.4 Asymmetric mentalis function noted during forceful eye closing. This is an example of synkinesis

with animation. Unusual patterns of dimples or wrinkles should be noticed, especially in the chin and mouth area (Fig. 11.4). Photography can also be useful in demonstrating subtle muscle abnormalities to patients.

Clinical Examples

Injury to the frontal branch of the facial nerve is one of the simplest areas to treat. Aggressive treatment of the contralateral frontalis and corrugator muscles will restore symmetry. The procerus may need treatment as well, although the zygomatic branch of the facial nerve running below the eye often innervates the procerus. Bilateral paralysis of the forehead is usually not perceptible at rest or in motion unless the patient has significant brow ptosis.

Asymmetry of ocular aperture is a fairly common occurrence. BTX-A can be used to counteract the 'big eye versus small eye.' The patient in Fig. 11.5 has subtle differences in ocular aperture; the right eye appears slightly smaller than the left eye and the discrepancy is accentuated when the patient is smiling (Fig. 11.6). Small dosages of BTX can be injected to improve symmetry. Generally 1–2 units are placed mid-pupillary line in the inferior orbicularis oculi muscle 1 mm from the cilliary margin (Fig. 11.7).

Another unappreciated asymmetry may be present in brow position. The patient in Fig. 11.3 has an elevated brow position on the right side. Correction can be achieved with the placement of more BTX on the right side of the frontalis muscle as compared to the left. To achieve symmetry, 6 units were administered to the right side and 4 units to the left. Brow asymmetry may also result from hyperfunction of the brow elevators to counteract eyelid ptosis. This is most commonly found in the older patient population. Treatment should be avoided, as this will exacerbate visual field problems (Figs 11.1 & 11.2).

The patient in Fig. 11.8 demonstrates a much more complex injury pattern. This patient suffered left-sided Bell's palsy 20 years before treatment. The facial nerve has regenerated in some areas to excess and not at all in other areas. The key to effective treatment is carefully to analyze muscles with excess function and others with deficient function.

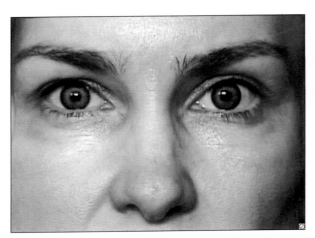

Fig. 11.5 Asymmetric eyes at rest, left eye is bigger than the right

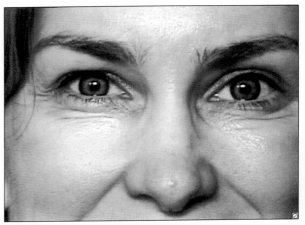

Fig. 11.6 Asymmetry is exacerbated with smiling

First, the face is examined at rest (Fig. 11.8). Each muscle group is assessed. The resting tone of the forehead is fairly symmetrical, with slight increased tone of the corrugator muscles. With animation, however, there is decreased function of the left frontalis muscle (Fig. 11.9). The corrugators are treated on both sides, as symmetry is easy to achieve with bilateral total muscle relaxation. A smaller dose is used on the left (regenerated) side as regenerated nerves seem to be more sensitive to BTX. The frontalis is treated only on the right (normal) side to achieve symmetry with animation. To avoid ptosis of the brow, the upper portion of the frontalis only is treated.

Next the eyes are examined. At rest, the left ocular aperture is smaller than the right, signaling hyperfunction of the regenerated pretarsal orbicularis muscle (Fig. 11.8). However, with animation, crow's feet are present on the patient's right (normal) side, but absent on the left (reinnervated) side (Fig. 11.10). This shows that the left lateral orbicularis is hypofunctional while the pretarsal portion of the same muscle is hyperfunctional. Thus a small amount of BTX is used on the left eye in the mid-pupillary line pretarsal orbicularis and a moderate amount is used on the right in the lateral orbicularis to decrease crow's feet. This combination produces enhanced symmetry at rest and in animation (Figs 11.11 and 11.12).

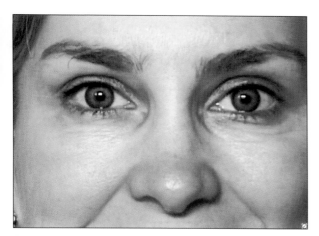

Fig. 11.7 BTX-A treatment to the crow's feet plus a single unit to the midline lower lid restores symmetry during smiling

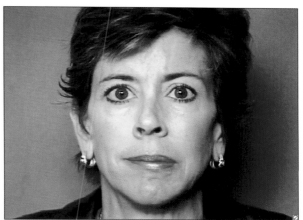

Fig. 11.8 Eighteen years after Bell's palsy on the left, several abnormalities are noted at rest

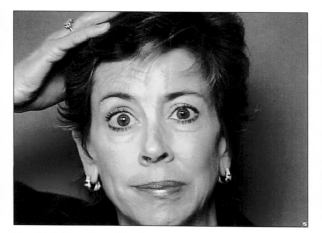

Fig. 11.9 Elevation of the brow reveals hypofunction of the left frontalis muscle

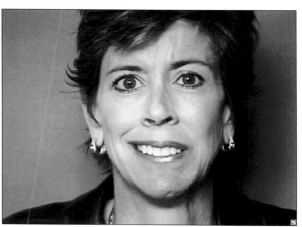

Fig. 11.10 Same patient, smiling highlights several asymmetries

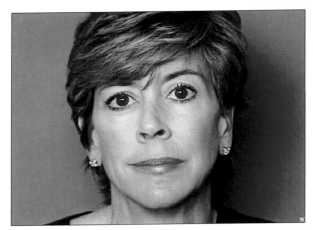

Fig. 11.11 After BTX-A therapy, perioral symmetry is enhanced at rest

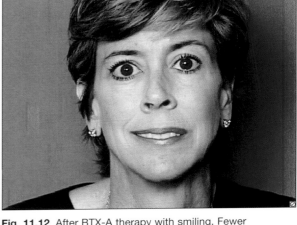

Fig. 11.12 After BTX-A therapy with smiling. Fewer asymmetries are noted

Examination of the mouth is challenging due to multiple muscles pulling in different directions. At rest, the left nasolabial fold is flat, signaling hypofunction of the levator muscles—levator labii superioris, levator anguli oris, zygomaticus major, and zygomaticus minor. The corner of the mouth is turned down, signifying relatively excessive function of the depressor labii inferioris and the depressor anguli oris. Also, at rest, dimpling of the mentalis muscle is present on the affected side, another sign of hyperfunction (Fig. 11.8). With animation, many of these asymmetries are amplified. The flattening of the nasolabial fold is more apparent, and the left upper lip is lower. Dimpling of the left mentalis is more pronounced, and chin lines from the depressor anguli oris are pronounced (Fig. 11.10).

Treatment of the mouth levators presents many difficulties. If attempted, doses need to be very small and overcorrection is common. This patient's left side weakness appears to be more zygomaticus major than levator, and treatment would be with 1–2 units of BTX in the origin of the zygomaticus major on the normal side, on the body of the zygoma. This patient chose not to have treatment of the upper mouth muscles. If excess function is more in the levator labii superioris aleque nasi, 1–2 units are placed just lateral to the piraform aperture. This injection site is also useful in softening the nasolabial folds in the patient with the 'gummy' smile, as the central lip drops.

Treatment of the depressor muscles of the mouth is simpler and more direct. Both the hyperfunctional side and the normal side are treated to ensure symmetry. The result is a lifting of the corner of the mouth and a smoothing of the chin. (Figs 11.11 and 11.12). This treatment improves perioral symmetry both at rest and in animation.

Discussion

BTX-A use has blossomed in several different fields as different indications are continually being discovered. Treatment of facial nerve irregularities is challenging, but allows a novel, minimally invasive treatment for very difficult problems. Like many therapies, there is a significant learning curve and novice users should certainly start with more straightforward cosmetic uses such as glabellar lines or crow's feet. The techniques described here are very difficult to master and require a careful analysis and understanding of underlying facial musculature.

Satisfied patients require a careful understanding of the ongoing nature of the treatment, its longevity, and the need for frequently administered adjustments. Knowing that each patient is unique, calculated trial and error will be necessary to optimize results.

Further Reading

Armstrong MWJ, Mountain RE, Murray JAM 1996 Treatment of facial synkinesis and facial asymmetry with botulinum toxin type A following facial nerve palsy. Clinical Otolaryngology 21:15–20

Biglan AW, May M, Bowers RA 1988 Management of facial spasm with *Clostridium botulinum* toxin, type A (Oculinum). Archives of Otolaryngological Head and Neck Surgery 114:1407–1412

Bikhazi HB, Maas CS 1997 Refinement in the rehabilitation of the paralyzed face using botulinum toxin. Otolaryngological Head and Neck Surgery 117(4):303–306

Campbell KE, Brundage JF 2002 Effects of climate, latitude, and season on the incidence of Bell's palsy in the US Armed Forces, October 1997 to September 1999. American Journal of Epidemiology 156(1):32–39

Clark RP, Berris CE 1989 Botulinum toxin: a treatment for facial asymmetry caused by facial nerve paralysis. Plastic and Reconstructive Surgery 84(2):353–355

Etkoff N 1999 Survival of the prettiest: the science of beauty. Random House, New York

May M, Shambaugh GE 1991 Facial nerve paralysis. In: Paparella MM, et al (eds) Otolaryngology. WB Saunders, Philadelphia, pp.1097–1136

Morris AM, Deeks SL, Hill MD, et al 2002 Annualized incidence and spectrum of illness from an outbreak investigation of Bell's palsy. Neuroepidemiology 21(5):255–261

Murray JAM 1992 Pathophysiology and assessment of the chronically paralyzed face. Facial Plastic Surgery 8(2):93–99

Tulley P, Webb A, Chana JS, et al 2000 Paralysis of the marginal mandibular branch of the facial nerve: treatment options. British Journal of Plastic Surgery 53:378–385

12 Complications of Cosmetic Botulinum Toxin Therapy

Anna Krishtul, Heidi A. Waldorf, Andrew Blitzer

Introduction

Injection of botulinum toxin (BTX) for treatment of hyperdynamic facial lines is a fast, relatively noninvasive procedure that produces significant esthetic improvement with minimal recovery downtime. Overwhelming patient satisfaction coupled with a rather mild side effect profile is generally responsible for the explosive popularity of esthetic use of BTX in the last decade. In a recent survey, 77% of patients treated with BTX for cosmetic indications expressed feeling more comfortable with their body, greater than 80% found the treatment beneficial, and all participants would recommend this therapy to others.

Years of experience have proven BTX to be safe and effective in the treatment of rhytides; nevertheless, discussion of complications of this treatment deserves attention. Because cosmetic use of BTX is entirely voluntary, significant adverse events are unacceptable. The complications associated with cosmetic use are uncommon, with the majority being mild and temporary, as is the therapeutic effect of the medication itself. To this day no serious or long-term side effects have been reported.

Because BTX-A has been available much longer than BTX-B, the bulk of scientific data published in the literature comes from studies with BTX-A. Although esthetic use of BTX-B has not been studied as extensively, its reported complications appear to be similar to those of BTX-A. Typically, the adverse events are related to the injection technique rather than the neurotoxin itself. As such, they are preventable with thorough knowledge of muscle anatomy and adequate training in technique. This chapter will list contraindications to BTX treatment, briefly review complications associated with its medical use, address proper patient selection, describe in detail adverse events reported with cosmetic use of BTX, and conclude with discussion of the issue of immunoresistance.

Contraindications

Absolute contraindications to BTX include known allergic reaction to any of the components in the formulation and pre-existing infection at the site of planned injection. In addition, practitioners should always clearly establish what kind of result the patient is expecting from this therapy. BTX should not be administered to patients with unrealistic expectations or any degree of hesitation regarding their decision to undergo this treatment. The manufacturer warns against using BTX in patients with known neuromuscular conditions, including diseases of the neuromuscular junction (e.g. myasthenia gravis and Lambert–Eaton syndrome) and peripheral motor neuropathies. BTX can worsen these neurologic conditions and cause serious systemic effects such as dysphagia and respiratory problems even when given at small doses. Additionally, presence of human albumin in BTX formulation carries a potential risk for transmission of viral diseases and Creutzfeldt–Jakob disease, although no cases have ever been reported.

Women who are lactating, pregnant or planning to become pregnant are not recommended to use BTX. The literature does not contain any reports of teratogenic effects of BTX; however, safety of this agent in pregnancy has not been established and it is currently classified as a category C drug. Likewise, nothing is known about excretion of BTX in breast milk; therefore, women should be advised to abstain from using it until their pregnancy is finished and they are no longer lactating.

Patients with inflammatory skin conditions (e.g. psoriasis, contact dermatitis, eczema) present

Contraindications to use of BTX	
Absolute contraindications	**Relative contraindications**
Hypersensitivity	Neuromuscular conditions
Infection at injection site	Concominant use of aminoglycosides, cholinesterase inhibitors, succinylcholine, curare-like depolarizing blockers, magnesium sulfate, quinidine, calcium channel blockers, lincosamides, polymyxins
	Pregnancy
	Lactation
	Inflammatory skin conditions
	Age > 65

Table 12.1 Contraindications to use of BTX

at the sites of proposed injections should not be using BTX until their condition is completely resolved. In addition, as BTX clinical trials did not include a sufficient number of patients over the age of 65, and especially over 75, the safety and efficacy of BTX in this age group has not been well studied. However, many practitioners regularly use BTX in the older patient population and will agree that this procedure may actually be more appropriate for a 70-year-old patient who had a facelift than a 60-year-old with significant redundant skin. A caveat to this is that physicians should be very cautious with patients who have undergone lower eyelid surgery as periocular use of BTX in these cases carries an increased risk of ectropion.

BTX should not be administered to patients taking certain medications due to potential drug interactions. Generally, these are medications known to interfere with neuromuscular transmission (e.g. aminoglycosides, cholinesterase inhibitors, succinyl-choline, curare-like depolarizing blockers, mag-nesium sulfate, quinidine, calcium channel blockers, lincosamides, polymyxins) (see Table 12.1).

Complications associated with medical use of BTX

Neurologists and ophthalmologists have long employed BTX for treatment of conditions related to muscle hyperactivity, including cervical and limb dystonia, spasmodic torticollis, hemifacial spasm, spasmodic dysphonia, cerebral palsy, blepharo-spasm, and strabismus. The typical therapeutic doses of BTX required for these indications are higher than those used for cosmetic procedures. Medical use of BTX has been well studied and publicized, providing us with a large body of

scientific data and clinical experience. Injection site pain, edema, erythema, and bruising are general adverse effects associated with the physical act of intramuscular injection itself. Idiosyncratic reactions like rash at a site distant to infection and anaphylaxis have been reported. Nausea, flu-like symptoms, and upper respiratory infection have all been described but their relationship to BTX is unclear. The majority of adverse events caused by BTX represent exten-sion of its therapeutic effect due to local and systemic toxin diffusion.

In patients with cervical dystonia, dysphagia, neck weakness, and dry mouth are the most com-mon complications of BTX therapy, with most cases being mild and self-limited. Overall incidence of dysphagia in patients treated with Botox® and Dysport® is 25–90%. In a study of Botox for treat-ment of cervical dystonia, 62% of participants reported mild dysphagia, 48% reported neck stiffness, 58% reported neck weakness, 61% reported pain at injec-tion site, and 18% reported flu-like symptoms. In studies with BTX-B (Neurobloc®), dysphagia was reported by 11–22%, dry mouth by 14–24%, with dose-related increase in incidence. Dry mouth is less frequently seen in patients using Botox than those using Dysport, and both cause less dry mouth than Neurobloc.

Short-lasting symptoms of dry eye are reported by up to 36% and ptosis by 14% of patients receiving BTX for treatment of blepharospasm. Occasional superficial punctuate keratitis and corneal erosions have also occurred. Ptosis and vertical deviation are major complications of BTX therapy in patients with strabismus. Frequency of induced ptosis ranges from 4 to 24%, with complete resolution within 6 weeks. Vertical deviation occurs in 8–60% and may persist for over a year in some cases.

Headache has been cited as a side effect of BTX therapy for strabismus and cervical dystonia, although it may be due to the act of injection itself. Interestingly, BTX has also been shown to be effective in treatment of chronic pain disorders, including headache. Published literature contains a number of studies demonstrating efficacy of BTX-A in relieving migraine, tension, and cervicogenic headache. The manufacturer of Botox describes rare reports of cardiovascular effects associated with noncosmetic use of BTX, including arrhythmia, hypertension, and myocardial infarction, some with fatal outcomes, although a causal relationship has not been established.

There are no published reports of localized weakness in muscles distant from BTX injection site in patients without an underlying neurological condition; however, single-fiber EMG studies have demonstrated subclinical changes in distant muscles. Iatrogenic botulism caused by therapeutic injections of BTX is exceedingly rare. Classic presentation of botulism includes symmetric descending flaccid paralysis with no changes in mental status. Three cases of generalized transient muscle weakness consistent with mild botulism have been reported following administration of therapeutic doses of BTX-A (Dysport) to patients with cervical dystonia. In addition, there are published reports of autonomic side effects of BTX, including dry mouth, accommodation difficulties, conjuctival irritation, and decreased sweating, which suggest systemic spread. It appears that BTX-B has a higher incidence of autonomic side effects than BTX-A. Diffusion is inversely proportional to molecular weight of a compound; therefore, systemic effects of BTX can be explained by rapid diffusion of its uncomplexed portion which has a rather low molecular weight of 150 kDa.

Long-term benefit and safety of BTX-A has been demonstrated by several studies involving patients with neurologic disorders. In a retrospective analysis of 235 patients who received a total of 2616 BTX-A treatment sessions for various movement disorders over a 10-year period, rate of side effects was 27% at any given time, occurring in only 4.5% of all sessions. Sustained treatment benefit was seen in 75.8% of patients for up to 10 years. Primary resistance developed in 9.1% of patients and secondary resistance in 7.5%, although serum antibody testing was not performed. It is interesting to note that only 1.3% of participants terminated therapy due to intolerable adverse effects.

Histological analysis of long-term intramuscular injections of BTX-A did not demonstrate any irreversible muscle atrophy or other degenerative changes. In addition, it has been shown that function of motor endplates returns to normal following BTX-A chemodenervation. Complications associated with cosmetic use of BTX will be discussed in detail later in the chapter.

Patient selection

Careful selection and screening of patients for any factors which might undermine the outcomes of BTX treatment is of outmost importance. The main goal of treatment should be patient satisfaction and avoidance of complications. Each potential candidate for BTX treatment must begin with a consultation visit during which the patient's goals and expectations are clearly delineated, questions are answered, and detailed medical history and focused physical exam are obtained.

Patient interview

Each patient should be thoroughly interviewed prior to receiving BTX treatment. To make this process more effective, a practitioner can create a standardized patient questionnaire and either mail it to the patient prior to their visit or have them fill it out in the office. Having a patient go through the questions beforehand not only saves time for a doctor and ensures that important information is not missed, but also forces the patient to think seriously about BTX treatment and analyze their own perceptions and expectations of this therapy. It is also a good idea to ask patients to bring a photo of themselves when they were younger or a photo of an older relative who looks like them. Such photos can be very useful for a physician to see how the patient's appearance has changed over the years and what other changes might take place.

Medical contraindications to BTX therapy have been discussed at the beginning of this chapter. In addition, certain psychosocial factors may have a negative impact on patients' satisfaction with treatment results. Any patient who is hesitant about BTX therapy or who has unrealistic expectations is a poor candidate for this procedure.

Physicians must also be very cautious with patients who have a history of psychiatric conditions. A patient who is mentally ill and expects BTX

Questions to ask patients

- Have you ever used BTX?
- Have you ever had any cosmetic procedures?
- Are you considering facial cosmetic surgery in the near future?
- What would you like to accomplish with BTX treatment?
- Do you have any conditions that might preclude you from using BTX (pregnancy or planning to become pregnant, breastfeeding, known allergy to BTX, neurological conditions, infection or inflammatory skin condition at the site for which treatment is desired)?
- Do you know how BTX works?
- Do you know that BTX treatment is a purely cosmetic procedure which is not covered by insurance and which requires regular injections every 3–4 months to maintain its effect?
- Are you allergic to any medications?
- List all oral and topical medications you are currently taking or have taken in the last month, including over-the-counter and herbal preparations.
- Past medical history, including easy bruising and bleeding, delayed wound healing, and predisposition to scar formation.
- Past surgical history, including cosmetic and eye-related surgery.
- Do you have any history of psychiatric conditions?
- Are you involved in any occupation where facial expressions are extremely important (e.g. acting, public speaking, politics)?
- Do you have any questions regarding BTX treatment?

Box 12.1 Questions to ask patients

treatment to make them feel better about themselves should be referred to a psychiatrist. Recently, a fascinating psychiatric entity has been reported called botulinophilia. This term is applied to patients with a body dysmorphic disorder who seek treatment with BTX. In one survey, 23% of patients requesting BTX for cosmetic indications were found to have this condition. Botulinophilia should be considered a contraindication to BTX treatment. These patients present a major challenge for a physician and will benefit from psychotherapy. Also, patients contemplating facial plastic surgery in the near future should be discouraged from treating their facial lines before the operation, unless, e.g. preoperative resetting of brow height or other indication would be a surgical advantage to the patient (Box 12.1).

Physical exam

A careful examination of the patient's face and neck is an essential component of the consultation visit. Good lighting and absence of makeup are very important for adequate assessment of facial lines. It is helpful to give patients a hand mirror and ask them to point out areas with which they are unhappy. Any signs of skin infection or inflammation, facial asymmetry, deep dermal scarring, and past facial surgery should be noted. Patients with thick sebaceous skin, redundant skin, as well as those with deep lines that do not improve significantly when the skin is physically stretched are poor candidates for BTX therapy. Beware of patients who had lower eyelid surgery as they are at a higher risk for developing ectropion after BTX treatment. A 'snap' test should be performed to assess the mobility of the eyelid. As well, patients with low-sitting foreheads and droopy upper eyelids are poor candidates for treatment of forehead rhytides because their eyelids may descend to the point of obstruction of their vision.

Complications associated with cosmetic use of BTX

Overall safety of BTX in doses used for cosmetic purposes is exceptional. Complications are uncommon, mild, and transient in nature. Irreversible clinical effects have never been reported with BTX. In clinical trials of Botox Cosmetic, 43.7% of treated subjects reported adverse effects of any type compared to 41.5% in placebo group, with headache, upper respiratory tract infection, blepharoptosis, nausea, pain, and flu-like symptoms being most common.

The majority of undesirable cosmetic outcomes are caused by improper injection technique and/or local diffusion of injected BTX which leads to weakness of adjacent muscles. Generally, the radius of neurotoxin diffusion is 1–3 cm measuring from the site of original injection. Reconstituting BTX with smaller amounts of diluent produces solution of higher concentration, thus requiring smaller volumes per injection. This approach translates into decreased local toxin spread and fewer side effects. Furthermore, most practitioners instruct their patients to stay upright for at least 4 hours following injections and avoid manipulation of the injected region, although the benefit of the former is debated.

General side effects

Adverse reactions related to the intramuscular injection itself include pain, erythema, edema, and bruising. Using smaller gauge needles and applying topical anesthetic prior to injection can significantly lessen the pain.

If anesthetic cream is to be used, patients should be advised to come in at least 30 minutes early because the medication requires time to take its full effect. Applying ice or cooling gel packs can also help reduce the discomfort as well as postinjection erythema and swelling. BTX-B (Myobloc) was reported as somewhat more painful than BTX-A, probably due to its acidic pH of 5.

Studies have also shown that reconstitution of both BTX-A and BTX-B with preservative-containing saline significantly reduces pain associated with injections when compared to BTX reconstituted with preservative-free saline. Importantly, no reduction in treatment efficacy was noted in these studies with up to 16 weeks' follow-up. Benzyl alcohol found in bacteriostatic saline is believed to be responsible for the anesthetic effect. To minimize postinjection bruising, patients should be instructed to abstain from aspirin for at least a week and nonsteroidal anti-inflammatory medications for several days prior to treatment. In addition, they should avoid vitamin E and herbal supplements with known blood-thinning properties such as ginseng, gingko, garlic, and ginger for 2 weeks. Patients taking prescription anticoagulants should consult their primary physician.

Idiosyncratic reactions such as headache, flu-like symptoms, respiratory tract infections, nausea, skin rash, pruritus, and allergic reaction have been reported. In a large randomized, placebo-controlled study of BTX-A (Botox) for glabellar rhytides, headache (BTX-A, 15.3%; placebo, 15%) and respiratory tract infection (BTX-A, 4.9%; placebo, 8.3%) were the most common complications, although no statistically significant differences among placebo and treatment groups were observed. The majority of reported cases were mild and transient, lasting only a few hours. In a smaller study of BTX-B (Myobloc) treatment for glabellar lines, 2.9% of patients experienced transient headache. Incidence of severe headache following treatment with BTX-A was 1% in one large series, with gradual resolution of symptoms after 2–4 weeks. No pre-disposing factors were identified. It has been hypothesized that the headache is caused by the muscle spasm produced by injected BTX. It is interesting to note that headache is not exclusively reported by patients who received injections to the face, but also to the palms for treatment of hyperhidrosis. In addition, BTX has been actually shown to be effective in treatment of various types of headache, most significantly migraine. All this evidence supports the conclusion that headache is most likely an idiosyncratic reaction to BTX injections. Patients suffering from postinjection headache should be treated with appropriate analgesics, including prescription medications if the pain is not relieved by usual over-the-counter agents.

Published literature contains a single case of a patient who developed metallic taste in her mouth after each treatment with BTX-A (Botox). This adverse reaction was self-limited and did not deter the patient from continuing BTX injections. When compared to placebo, cosmetic use of BTX-A has not been associated with significant changes in blood pressure and heart rate or standard blood counts and chemistry.

Forehead

Brow ptosis is the most important complication of forehead rhytide treatment (Fig. 12.1). Because the lower 2.5–4 cm of frontalis is responsible for brow movement, paralysis of this muscle can bring the eyebrows down, especially in a patient with a low forehead. Older patients with redundant skin under the eyebrow are also at risk for pseudo-ptosis. Careful patient selection and avoidance of BTX injections above the middle brow or within 1 cm of the bony supraorbital margin will decrease the risk of brow ptosis. As the brow location and appearance can be altered, direct palpation of the orbital edge is a more reliable method of establishing a point of reference. Brow ptosis can also be partially mitigated by injecting brow depressors. Some physicians discourage injections of frontalis alone and recommend concomitant injection of frontalis and brow depressors, particularly in patients over 50 and those with low-set eyebrows and pre-existing brow ptosis. However, this maneuver can immobilize the entire eyebrow and cause a lack of expression. Combined injection of the glabella and forehead should be done with caution as it carries a very high risk of brow ptosis.

Another, less common, complication seen with treatment of frontal lines is upper eyelid ptosis (Fig. 12.2). It is usually induced by downward diffusion of neurotoxin into the eyelid levator muscle following injection of BTX at or above the

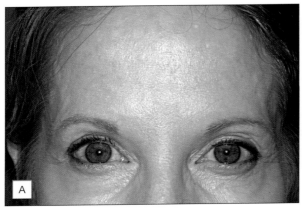
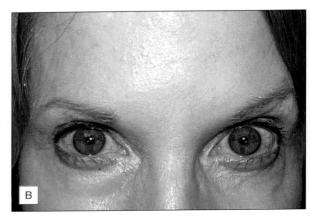

Fig. 12.1 (**A**) Pre-BTX-A injection to glabella and frontalis. (**B**) Post-BTX-A injection showing lowered central eyebrows and marked left lateral eyebrow elevation (Courtesy of A. and J. Carruthers, MD)

eyebrow at midpupillary line. Patients who rely on frontalis muscle to help elevate their eyelids are especially at risk for secondary upper eyelid ptosis. If such a complication does occur, patients should be given eye drops containing α-adrenergic agonists, e.g. apraclonidine (Iopidine; Alcon Laboratories, Fort Worth, TX, USA) or phenylephrine (Neosynephrine hydrochloride, 2.5%; Sanofi, Winthrop Pharmaceuticals New York) to apply to the affected eye as needed until the symptoms resolve. These two agents can help elevate the upper lid by contracting Muller's muscle which is adrenergically innervated.

Finally, inadequate weakening of the lateral portion of frontalis muscle will produce lateral arching of the brow, creating a 'cocked' or 'Jack Nicholson' appearance (Fig. 12.1). This cosmetically unappealing effect can be reduced by injecting a small amount of BTX into the lateral frontalis.

Glabella

Ptosis of the upper eyelid is the most significant complication seen with treatment of glabellar wrinkles. In one large study with BTX-A (Botox), the incidence of blepharoptosis following glabella injections was 5.4%, with most cases being mild. In another, smaller study with BTX-B (Myobloc), 5.9% of patients developed this complication. Improper injection technique such as placing BTX too close to the upper bony orbital rim can produce this effect. It may take anywhere from 48 hours to 2 weeks for ptosis to develop and it can persist for 2–4 weeks or even longer, occasionally. Again, diffusion of the neurotoxin is responsible for this

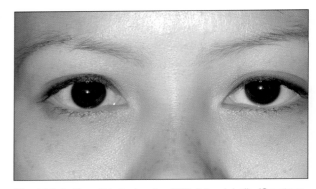

Fig. 12.2 Left eyelid ptosis after BTX-A to glabella (Courtesy of A. and J. Carruthers, MD)

unfavorable outcome. Some physicians recommend applying digital pressure at the supraorbital border during corrugator injections in order to decrease BTX diffusion. Similarly to frontalis injections, one should avoid placing BTX closer than 1 cm above the bony supraorbital margin above the upper lid levator, i.e. between the medial and lateral canthi. Symptomatic treatment of eyelid ptosis has been described in the preceding section.

Periocular area

The most common complication of crow's feet treatment is bruising secondary to the rich vascular supply and thin skin characteristic of this region. Orbicularis oculi is a thin muscle, therefore superficial injections can minimize bruising without loss of efficacy. In addition, placing each injection at the advancing edge of the previous one, forming a wheal, helps avoid disruption of blood vessels and decreases the risk of bruising (Fig. 12.3). Generous ice application is also beneficial.

Specific side effects related to injection of BTX for treatment of crow's feet include diplopia, loss of voluntary eye closure, and upper lip ptosis. Diplopia and loss of voluntary eye closure can be avoided by injecting BTX at least 1 cm lateral to the orbital rim or 1.5 cm from the lateral canthus. BTX injected too close to the lateral canthus may diffuse medially and cause weakness of the lateral rectus muscle with resulting horizontal diplopia, although it is rare. Patients who develop this complication should be referred to an ophthalmologist skilled in the use of BTX and instructed to temporarily cover the affected eye to help with double vision.

Paralysis of the palpebral segment of orbicularis oculi muscle is responsible for the loss of voluntary eye closure. General recommendations for managing this adverse effect include taping the affected eye shut during the night and application of moisturizing eye drops. Placing an injection too close to the inferior border of the zygomatic arch or too deep will weaken the zygomaticus major muscle and produce upper lip ptosis, similar to Bell's palsy. Zygomaticus major is adjacent to the orbicularis oculi muscle and is an important upper lip elevator. In one study, estimated incidence of this complication was 0.3% per pair or 0.15% per side. The authors of this study reported on three cases which, interestingly, all occurred in patients who had undergone facial plastic surgery.

Altered periocular anatomy was speculated to be the cause of unexpected BTX diffusion. Upper lip ptosis can last up to 6 weeks, which is longer than most other complications and has no treatment. Finally, injection too close to the lateral canthus can cause atrophy in the muscle in this area, making the lateral part of orbicularis oculi more obvious and causing a significant cosmetic defect (Fig. 12.4).

Injection of the hypertrophied lower pretarsal portion of orbicularis to widen the palpebral aperture has been associated with ectropion and dry eye (keratoconjuctivitis sicca). To prevent dry eye, the BTX dose should be limited to 2 units. Ectropion is caused by paralysis of the inferior portion of the orbicularis oculi muscle and this may also cause excessive scleral show inferiorly (Fig. 12.5). Three groups of patients are particularly at risk for this complication: those with redundant infraorbital skin (can be confirmed with a snap test, i.e. lower eyelid slowly returns to its original position when it is pulled down), those with significant pre-existing scleral show, and those who have had lower eyelid surgery.

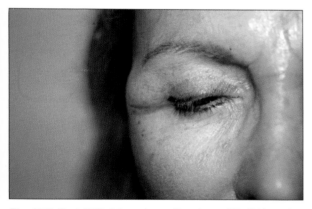

Fig. 12.3 Post-BTX-A hematoma (Courtesy of Dr D.Hexsel)

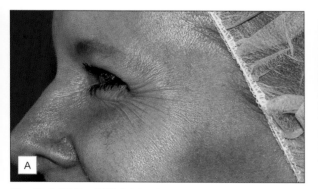

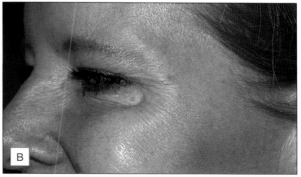

Fig. 12.4 (A) Pre-BTX-A injection to crow's feet and infraorbital orbicularis. (B) Postinjection too close to the canthus showing muscle atrophy (Courtesy of A. and J. Carruthers, MD)

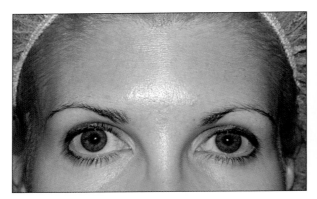

Fig. 12.5 Scleral show after too aggressive use of BTX-A in the lower eyelid (Courtesy of A. and J. Carruthers, MD)

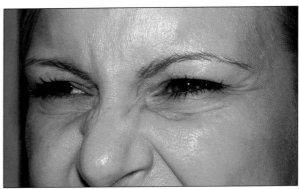

Fig. 12.6 Exaggeration of the scrunch lines after glabella BTX-A: the Botox sign (Courtesy of A. and J. Carruthers, MD)

Festooning of the lower orbital skin has been reported after infraorbital injection with BTX-A in a patient with prior lower lid blepharoplasty. Complete resolution occurred within 3–4 weeks after treatment. Disruption of the infraorbital portion of orbicularis oculi muscle during surgery may have weakened the muscle enough to cause this complication after further muscle weakening with BTX injection. There has also been a report of orbital fat herniation in a patient treated with BTX for crow's feet. The deformity persisted for 5 months. The orbicularis oculi muscle is partially responsible for integrity of the inferior fat pad, which can herniate when the inferior aspect of this muscle is weakened.

Mid and lower face

BTX must be used with caution in the mid and lower face due to highly variable muscular anatomy. Generally, lower doses are employed compared to the upper face. Treatment of 'bunny lines' (Fig. 12.6), fine smile lines that are caused by contraction of upper nasalis muscle and radiate medially from the dorsum of the nose, can be complicated by ipsilateral lip ptosis secondary to weakening of levator labii superioris. To prevent this complication, injection should be placed high on the lateral nasal wall, well above the nasofacial groove. Furthermore, vigorous or downward postinjection massage should be avoided to prevent undesirable neurotoxin diffusion.

Injecting depressor septae muscle for treatment of nasal tip droop can cause upper lip ptosis. Patients who naturally have a long nonvermilion upper lip are especially at risk for unsatisfactory esthetic outcome and should be approached with caution.

Treatment of nasolabial folds with BTX has not been very successful and soft tissue fillers remain the mainstream treatment for this area. Experience has showed that injections into levator labii superioris alaeque nasi causes lengthening of the upper lip, which only accentuates the aging facial changes. In addition, this procedure can be complicated by upper lip ptosis and smile asymmetry. The only patients who may benefit from this approach are those with short upper lips.

The perioral area should be approached with caution to prevent an incompetent mouth. When injecting orbicularis oris for effacement of vertical lip lines, care must be taken to place small doses of BTX superficially and symmetrically in relation to the midline. Weakening of the lip sphincter, which may be asymmetric (Fig. 12.7), is a side effect associated with this procedure. Rarely, it can be significant enough to impair the patient's ability to pucker, whistle, drink from a straw, put on lipstick, kiss, pronounce 'p' and 's' sounds, and play wind musical instruments. Patients whose occupations require full function of this area, e.g. musicians, speakers, and singers, should be counseled prior to the procedure. In addition, injecting certain perioral areas should be avoided altogether. Lateral lip ptosis and drooling can occur due to weakening of lateral lip elevators with injections at the corners of the mouth. Upper lip midline injection can cause flattening of the cupid's bow.

Some physicians have injected BTX directly into depressor anguli oris muscle to alleviate the unpleasant downward deflection of the corner of

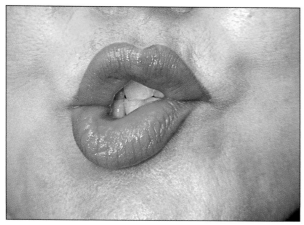

Fig. 12.7 Asymmetric lower lip following perioral BTX-A injection (Courtesy of A. and J. Carruthers, MD)

the mouth. Injecting too close to the mouth can produce a flaccid cheek, an incompetent mouth, and asymmetric smile. When treating melomental folds ('drool grooves' or marionette lines), BTX should be injected low at the junction of the depressor labii and inferior border of the mandible. Ipsilateral weakness of the depressor labii leading to flattening of the lower lip can be produced by injecting too medially. On the other hand, too high an injection can cause weakness of the lip sphincter with resulting impaired speech and suction movement. Combination of BTX and soft tissue fillers is the most effective treatment approach to this area. Injection of BTX into mentalis can soften the mental crease and improve the appearance of peau d'orange chin ('orange peel' dimpling). To avoid weakening of orbicularis oris with subsequent incompetent mouth, the mentalis injection must be placed at the most distal point from the orbicularis oris.

Bilateral injections into the levator labii superioris muscle have been used to correct the upper gum show during smiling. This procedure can be complicated by vertical elongation of the upper lip, which is a part of the normal aging process. Therefore, this treatment is not recommended for older patients.

Neck

BTX has been successfully used to treat vertical platysmal bands. Care must be taken not to inject too deep and use the lowest effective doses of the neurotoxin. Diffusion or direct injection of BTX into the underlying sternocleidomastoid and laryngeal muscles can produce dysphagia, change of voice pitch, and weakness of neck flexors. Maximum recommended dose of BTX ranges from 30 to 100 U/session. Patients with significant loss of cervical skin elasticity and fat descent are poor candidates for this procedure and would obtain better cosmetic results with rhytidectomy surgery. When treating horizontal neck lines, superficial injections of small doses of BTX will prevent inadvertent involvement of laryngeal muscles and excessive bruising due to disruption of deeper venous perforators, particularly in lateral aspects of the neck.

Hyperhidrosis

Temporary weakness of intrinsic muscles of the hand is a common complication of BTX treatment of palmar hyperhidrosis. It is caused by local diffusion of the neurotoxin. In a 3-year follow-up study of patients treated with BTX-A (Dysport), nine of 21 participants developed mild, transient reduction in finger power (measured by a strength test), lasting 4–8 weeks, with a mean duration of 5.7 weeks. In another study of 37 patients injected with BTX-A (Botox), 74% reported subjective hand weakness; nevertheless, 91% of patients wanted to continue treatment with the same dose of BTX. In all participants, neurophysiological testing demonstrated a decrease in compound muscle action potential for both abductor pollicis brevis and abductor digiti minimi by 64 and 36%, respectively, with normalization at 37 weeks. Abnormalities in neuromuscular transmission were detected on repetitive nerve stimulation and single fiber EMG. Sensory function remained unaffected. Interestingly, subjective muscle weakness did not correlate with objective measurements, therefore, physicians should be aware of subclinical weakness. To decrease the risk of this complication, it is generally recommended to inject BTX superficially and treat only one hand at a time to avoid bilateral hand weakness, which could be more difficult for a patient to tolerate. Patients whose occupations rely on intricate manual work, e.g. musicians, jewelers, and surgeons should be carefully counseled prior to this procedure.

BTX-A (Dysport) treatment of axillary hyperhidrosis has been associated with transient, local postinjection itching, and compensatory sweating in other areas with a mean duration of 12 weeks. None of these side effects were serious enough to deter patients from further treatment. There are two reported cases of systemic botulism-like syndrome following BTX injections for treatment of hyperhidrosis. In one case, a 25-year old female developed signs of systemic cholinergic impairment and generalized muscle weakness, including bilateral ptosis, diplopia, finger muscle weakness, diffuse asthenia, and decreased sweating, salivary production, and lacrimation 6 days after receiving BTX-A (Dysport) for concomitant treatment of axillary and palmar hyperhidrosis (total dose 1400 U). Single-fiber EMG revealed pathological jitters characteristic of neuromuscular transmission failure. Complete recovery occurred after 2 months. The other case involved a 27-year-old male patient with palmar hyperhidrosis who developed bilateral blurred vision, indigestion, and a dry throat with resulting dysphagia 2 days after BTX-B (Myobloc) injections (total 5000 U). His symptoms fully resolved after 3 weeks.

To reduce the risk of systemic side effects, lowest effective doses should be used. In addition, patients with multiple affected areas should have their treatments performed at different sessions to decrease the total dose of BTX.

Immunoresistance

The explosive popularity of BTX therapy raises the serious issue of immunoresistance to the neurotoxin. There are eight known serotypes of bacterium *Clostridium botulinum*, with seven serologically different neurotoxins. Each of these toxins has a unique binding site on the cell membrane and a distinct intracellular site of action. Repetitive injections of BTX can lead to formation of neutralizing

antibodies against that particular neurotoxin. Clinically, presence of such antibodies translates into a diminished or absent therapeutic response. In one long-term, retrospective study of 235 patients treated with BTX-A for various movement disorders, 9.1% of patients developed primary resistance (defined as less than 25% improvement after two to three trials with escalating doses of neurotoxin) and 7.5% developed secondary resistance (defined as less than 50% improvement for at least two cycles followed by less than 25% improvement after two or more subsequent cycles), which was similar to other studies. Antigenicity of BTX has been linked to the amount of protein complexed with the neurotoxin.

The original bulk of Botox (lot 79/11) produced by Allergan Inc. until 1998 contained 25 ng protein/100 U neurotoxin. Subsequently, protein load was decreased to 5 ng/100 U (Table 12.2).

The incidence of immunoresistance to BTX cited in the literature is largely based on older batches of BTX-A. In a recent study involving 130 cervical dystonia patients, neutralizing antibodies were found in 9.5% of patients treated with the original BTX-A compared to 0% in those treated with current neurotoxin. Both preparations had similar efficacy and side effect profile.

Immunoresistance has also been an issue with BTX-B. In a study of 446 patients with cervical dystonia, incidence of neutralizing antibodies was projected to be 18% after 18 months of treatment. It appears that the development of resistance is related to treatment dose and interval between injections rather than the total dose of BTX. Patients resistant to BTX-A have been shown to respond to treatments with BTX-B. There have been reports of cross-reactivity between different BTX

Protein load per 100 U and clinical equivalence of different BTX preparations		
BTX preparation	**Protein load per 100 U**	**Clinical equivalence**
Original Botox (BTX-A)	25 ng	1 U
Current Botox (BTX-A)	5 ng	1 U
Dysport (BTX-A)	2.5 ng	2.5–5 U
Myobloc/Neurobloc (BTX-B)	1 ng	50–100 U

Table 12.2 Protein load per 100 U and clinical equivalence of different BTX preparations

serotypes. Some Botox-resistant patients were found to have antibodies not only against BTX-A but also against BTX-B without ever being exposed to it. Marked homology between serotypes can explain such cross-reactivity. It is also possible that antibodies to one serotype can neutralize neurotoxin of another serotype.

Because doses of BTX used for cosmetic purposes are much smaller compared to those used for some medical indications, the risk of immunoresistance is greatly decreased. Indeed, the incidence of neutralizing antibodies with esthetic use is estimated at 1–2%, which does not always correlate with clinical effect. Nevertheless, BTX-B is still a viable option for those few who become unresponsive to BTX-A. In a recent study, 20 patients refractory to BTX-A had their glabellar rhytides successfully treated with BTX-B (Myobloc), although these individuals were not truly immunoresistant to BTX-A.

In summary, using the lowest possible effective dose of neurotoxin at each session and spacing treatments as far as possible are key in prevention of immunoresistance and maintainance of the long-term benefit of BTX.

Further Reading

Alam M, Arndt K, Dover J 2002 Severe, intractable headache after injection with botulinum A exotoxin: report of five cases. Journal of the American Academy of Dermatology 46:62–65

Alam M, Dover J, Arndt K 2002 Pain associated with injection of botulinum A exotoxin reconstituted using saline with and without preservative: a double-blind, randomized controlled trial. Archives of Dermatology 38:510–514

Alam M, Dover J, Klein A, et al 2002 Botulinum A exotoxin for hyperfunctional facial lines. Archives of Dermatology 138:1180–1185

Aoki K 1999 Preclinical update of Botox (botulinum toxin type A)-purified neurotoxin complex relative to other botulinum neurotoxin preparations. European Journal of Neurology 6(Suppl 4):S3–10

Bhatia K, Munchau A, Thompson P, et al 1999 Generalized muscular weakness after botulinum toxin injections for dystonia: a report of three cases. Journal of Neurological Neurosurgery in Psychiatry 67:90–93

Borodic G, Ferrante R 1992 Effects of repeated botulinum toxin injections on orbicularis oculi muscle. Journal of Clinical Neuroophthalmology 12:121–127

Botox Cosmetic monograph 2002. Allergan Inc., Irvine, CA, USA.

Brashear A, Bergan K, Wojcieszek J, et al 2000 Patients' perception of stopping or continuing treatment of cervical dystonia with botulinum toxin type A. Movement Disorders 15(1):150–153

Brashear A, Lew M, Dykstra D, et al 1999 Safety and efficacy of Neurobloc (botulinum toxin type B) in type A-responsive cervical dystonia. Neurology 53:1439–1446

Brin M, Lew M, Adler C, et al 1999 Safety and efficacy of Neurobloc (botulinum toxin type B) in type A-resistant cervical dystonia. Neurology 53:1431–1438

Carruthers A, Carruthers J 2000 Toxins 99, new information about the botulinum neurotoxins. Dermatological Surgery 26:174–176

Carruthers A, Lowe N, Menter A, et al 2002 A multicenter, double-blind, randomized, placebo-controlled study of the efficacy and safety of botulinum toxin type A in the treatment of glabellar lines. Journal of the American Academy of Dermatology 46:840–849

Carruthers J, Carruthers A 2003 Aesthetic botulinum A toxin in the mid and lower face. Dermatological Surgery 29:468–476

Comella C 2002 Cervical dystonia: treatment with botulinum toxin serotype A as Botox® or Dysport®. In: Brin M, Jankovic J, Hallett M (eds) Scientific and therapeutic aspects of botulinum toxin. Lippincott Williams & Wilkins, Philadelphia, p.362

Defazio G, Abbruzzesse G, Girlanda P, et al 2002 Botulinum toxin A treatment for primary hemifacial spasm: a 10-year multicenter study. Archives of Neurology 59:418–420

Dressler D, Benecke R 2003 Autonomic side effects of botulinum toxin type B treatment of cervical dystonia and hyperhidrosis. European Neurology 49:34–38

Goldman M 2003 Festoon formation after infraorbital botulinum A toxin: a case report. Dermatological Surgery 29:560–561

Harth W, Linse R 2001 Botulinophilia: contraindication for therapy with botulinum toxin. International Journal of Clinical Pharmacology and Therapeutics 39(10):460–463

Hsiung G-Y, Das S, Ranaway R, et al 2002 Long-term efficacy of botulinum toxin A in the treatment of various disorders over a 10-year period. Movement Disorders 17(6):1288–1293

Jankovic J 2002 Botulinum toxin: clinical implications of antigenicity and immunoresistance. In: Brin M, Jankovic J, Hallett M (eds) Scientific and therapeutic aspects of botulinum toxin. Lippincott Williams & Wilkins, Philadelphia, p.413

Jankovic J, Vuong K, Ahsan J 2003 Comparison of efficacy and immunogenicity of original versus current botulinum toxin in cervical dystonia. Neurology 60:1186–1188

Klein A 2003 Complications, adverse reactions, and insights with the use of botulinum toxin. Dermatological Surgery 29:549–556

Matarasso S, Matarasso A 2001 Treatment guidelines for botulinum toxin type A for the periocular region and a report on partial upper lip ptosis following injections to the lateral canthal rhytids. Plastic and Reconstructive Surgery 108:208–214

Matarasso S 2003 Comparison of botulinum toxin types A and B: a bilateral and double-blind randomized evaluation in the treatment of canthal rhytids. Dermatological Surgery 29:7–13

Mauriello J 2002 The role of botulinum toxin type A (Botox®) in the management of blepharospasm and hemifacial spasm. In: Brin M, Jankovic J, Hallett M (eds) Scientific and therapeutic aspects of botulinum toxin. Lippincott Williams & Wilkins, Philadelphia, p.201

Murray C, Solish N 2003 Metallic taste: an unusual reaction to botulinum toxin A. Dermatological Surgery 29:562–563

Myobloc monograph 2000, Elan Pharmaceuticals, Inc., San Francisco, CA, USA.

Paloma V, Samper A 2001 A complication with the aesthetic use of Botox: herniation of the orbital fat. Plastic and Reconstructive Surgery 107:1315–1317

Racette B, Lopate G, Good L, et al 2002 Ptosis as a remote effect of therapeutic botulinum toxin B injection. Neurology 59:1445–1447

Ramirez A, Reeck J, Maas C 2002 Botulinum toxin B (Myobloc) in the management of hyperkinetic facial lines. Otolaryngological Head and Neck Surgery 126:459–467

Schnider P, Moraru E, Kittler H, et al 2001 Treatment of focal hyperhidrosis with botulinum toxin type A: long-term follow-up in 61 patients. British Journal of Dermatology 145:289–293

Sommer B, Zschocke I, Bergfeld D, et al 2003 Satisfaction of patients after treatment with botulinum toxin for dynamic facial lines. Dermatological Surgery 29:456–460

Swartling C, Färnstrand C, Abt G, et al 2001 Side effects of intradermal injections of botulinum A toxin in the treatment of palmar hyperhidrosis: a neurophysiological study. European Journal of Neurology 8:451–456

Tugnoli V, Eleopra R, Quatrale R, et al 2002 Botulism-like syndrome after botulinum toxin type A injections for focal hyperhidrosis. British Journal of Dermatology 147:808–809

Wilson F 2001 Botulinum toxin-A risks overcome by proper technique. Cosmetic Surgery Times March:12

Subject Index

ELSEVIER DVD-ROM LICENSE AGREEMENT